Alan Bradley

Personal Alchemy
The Art of Self-Transformation

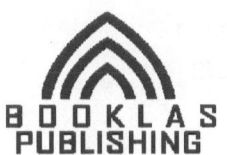

Original Title: *Personal Alchemy*
Copyright © 2024 by Luiz Antonio dos Santos
All rights reserved to Booklas Publishing
This book is intended for personal and spiritual development. The information and practices described are grounded in research, traditional wisdom, and the experiences of authors and experts in the field. It is not a substitute for medical advice or conventional therapies, but a complementary resource for well-being and personal growth.

Production Team
Editor: Luiz Antonio dos Santos
Text Revision: João Fernandes, Beatriz Lima
Graphic Design and Layout: Helena Castro
Cover Design: Booklas Studio / Lucas Silva

Publication Details
Personal Alchemy/ By Luiz Antonio dos Santos
Booklas Publishing, 2024
Categories: Personal Development. Spirituality. Holism.
I. Silva, Lucas. II. Castro, Helena. III. Title.
DDC: 158.1 - **CDU:** 159.9

Rights Reserved
Booklas Publishing
José Delalíbera Street, 962
86.183-550 – Cambé – PR
Email: support@booklas.com
Website: www.booklas.com

Sumário

Prologue 5
Chapter 1 Fundamentals of Transformation 7
Chapter 2 The Power of Now 11
Chapter 3 Mapping the Mind 15
Chapter 4 Limiting Beliefs 19
Chapter 5 Reframing 23
Chapter 6 Resource States 27
Chapter 7 Identifying Patterns 31
Chapter 8 Transformative Language 35
Chapter 9 The Inner Mirror 39
Chapter 10 Creative Visualization 43
Chapter 11 Conscious Communication 47
Chapter 12 The Power of Empathy 51
Chapter 13 Positive Anchors 54
Chapter 14 State Breaking 58
Chapter 15 Self-Responsibility 62
Chapter 16 Values and Purpose 66
Chapter 17 Focus and Direction 70
Chapter 18 Emotional Detachment 74
Chapter 19 Mirroring Technique 78
Chapter 20 Emotional Intelligence 82
Chapter 21 Overcoming Fear 86
Chapter 22 The Power of Gratitude 90
Chapter 23 Self-Sabotage 94
Chapter 24 Mental Reprogramming 98

Chapter 25 Internal Communication 102
Chapter 26 Relaxation Techniques 106
Chapter 27 Reframing Trauma 110
Chapter 28 Modeling Excellence 114
Chapter 29 Internal Alignment 118
Chapter 30 Mental Resilience 122
Chapter 31 Breaking Limits 126
Chapter 32 Body Language 130
Chapter 33 The Cycle of Change 134
Chapter 34 The Power of Feedback 138
Chapter 35 Emotions as Guides 142
Chapter 36 Habit Transformation 146
Chapter 37 Expanding Perception 150
Chapter 38 The Flow of Life 154
Chapter 39 Affirmation Techniques 158
Chapter 40 Assertive Communication 162
Chapter 41 Time as an Ally 166
Chapter 42 The Practice of Silence 170
Chapter 43 Perspective Shifting 174
Chapter 44 The Subconscious 178
Chapter 45 Strengthening Self-Confidence 182
Chapter 46 The Art of Forgiveness 186
Chapter 47 Overcoming Procrastination 190
Chapter 48 Celebrating Achievements 194
Chapter 49 Building Connections 198
Epilogue 202

Prologue

There is a hidden invitation within the pages now in your hands. This book is not merely a collection of words but a silent call to something greater: a journey that touches the roots of who you are and unveils the potential of who you can become. By opening these pages, you are not simply beginning a reading experience but crossing a threshold that few dare to traverse.

Within you lies a dormant alchemist, a creator capable of transforming the ordinary into the extraordinary, chaos into harmony, and the unknown into wisdom. This is not about distant magic or secrets reserved for the privileged few. It is about an inner science, a dance between the mind and the soul that, when aligned, can reshape every aspect of your life.

The words that follow are not mere explanations; they are keys. Each concept is a door to transformation, each practice a map to uncharted territory. Here, there are no impositions or absolute truths. There are tools, ideas, and pathways. The power lies in you—in your choices, in your courage to see the familiar with new eyes and the unfamiliar with curiosity.

Have you ever felt that there is something more, a deeper layer beneath the surface of daily experiences? That your patterns, challenges, and even triumphs carry messages you have yet to decipher? This book is a guide to decoding those signals, embracing the power to reframe, recreate, and transcend.

Every page is imbued with intention. The practices described are not mere exercises but portals to an expanded state of awareness. They are invitations for you to become the architect of your own story, the author of a destiny shaped by conscious choices rather than automatic reactions. The alchemy proposed here is not esoteric; it is practical, real, and rooted in neuroscience, ancient wisdom, and human experience.

As you read, feel the words as if they were written directly for you. Because, indeed, they are. This book is a mirror, reflecting not only who you are but who you can become. It speaks to that part of you that knows there is something more, that feels the pulse of a greater purpose. With each line, allow yourself to open to the possibilities. Each concept is a seed. It is up to you to cultivate it, nurture it, and witness how it flourishes in your life.

There are no coincidences. If these words have reached you, it is because you are ready to receive them. The world you have known so far does not have to be the limit. There are deeper layers of understanding, higher levels of achievement, and an abundance of inner resources waiting to be discovered.

As you delve into this book, you are accepting a pact with yourself: the commitment to grow, to challenge yourself, to transform. And at the end of this journey, you may discover that what you were truly searching for was not a new you, but the essence of who you have always been. Welcome to your own alchemy.

Chapter 1
Fundamentals of Transformation

Transformation begins in the quiet corners of our minds, where thoughts emerge, shapeless and endless, forming the essence of who we are. It is here, amidst the labyrinth of beliefs and behaviors, that change first takes root. To reshape oneself is to embark on a journey that transcends mere adjustment—it is alchemy, a process of profound metamorphosis that turns the raw elements of one's life into a masterpiece of personal evolution.

Personal Alchemy, as it is called, embodies this art of transformation. It is not a fleeting change but a deep reworking of the self, grounded in the understanding that the life we experience is an intricate dance of perception and response. Through this lens, every belief, every pattern, becomes a key, unlocking the potential to create a new reality.

The essence of this process lies in recognizing the interconnectedness of our thoughts, emotions, and actions. Each belief we hold, whether empowering or limiting, shapes the framework through which we interpret the world. These beliefs become habits of thought, repeating until they etch pathways in our minds. Behaviors follow, automatic and ingrained, forming the rhythm of our daily existence. To change, one must first understand this rhythm.

This is where the practice of Neuro-Linguistic Programming (NLP) offers its guidance. Rooted in the exploration of human cognition and communication, NLP is a toolkit for understanding and altering the mental patterns that govern behavior. It provides practical strategies to deconstruct the structures of our minds and rebuild them with intention and clarity.

NLP begins with the premise that the map is not the territory. This means that the way we perceive reality is a subjective construction, shaped by our experiences, beliefs, and biases. By understanding this, one gains the power to reshape their internal map, altering their perception of the world and their place within it.

Beliefs are among the first aspects to be explored. They act as invisible architects, building the walls that define what we consider possible. For instance, a person who believes they are unworthy of success will unconsciously avoid opportunities that might challenge this belief. The belief, self-perpetuating, becomes a prison. But when exposed to scrutiny, such beliefs often crumble. NLP teaches techniques to question these assumptions, revealing their fragility and opening the way for new, empowering convictions to take root.

Behaviors, too, must be examined. Each action, no matter how insignificant it seems, contributes to the mosaic of our lives. Habits form as neural pathways deepen with repetition, creating a default mode of operation. NLP's methods focus on interrupting these patterns, introducing new choices that align with the desired transformation.

One powerful tool within this realm is the anchoring technique. This involves associating a specific stimulus with a positive emotional state. For example, recalling a moment of confidence while performing a physical gesture, such as pressing two fingers together, can create a connection between the gesture and the emotion. Over time, this anchor can be used to evoke the desired state at will, helping to rewire habitual responses.

Personal transformation also requires a commitment to self-awareness. This means cultivating the ability to observe oneself without judgment, a practice that many find challenging. The mind resists scrutiny, protecting its habits and patterns from change. Yet, it is through this practice of observation that one begins to see the threads of their own narrative, unraveling the stories that no longer serve them.

As these threads are pulled apart, one begins to weave a new story, one that aligns with their true potential. This process requires courage, for transformation is not always comfortable. The familiar, even when painful, often feels safer than the unknown. But in embracing the discomfort of change, one discovers a freedom that transcends fear.

A central concept in Personal Alchemy is the power of choice. Every moment presents an opportunity to choose differently, to step away from the old patterns and create something new. This is not a matter of willpower alone but of clarity—knowing what one truly desires and aligning their actions with that vision. NLP emphasizes this alignment, teaching techniques to clarify goals and break them into actionable steps.

Another cornerstone of transformation is the recognition of interconnectedness—not only within oneself but also with the world around. As the internal shifts, so does the external. Relationships, environments, and circumstances begin to reflect the changes within, creating a ripple effect that extends far beyond the individual.

To embark on this journey of transformation is to accept the duality of destruction and creation. The old must be dismantled to make way for the new. This is not a linear process but a cycle, one that repeats as deeper layers of the self are uncovered and refined. It requires patience and persistence, for true change is seldom instant.

Throughout this chapter, the foundation of transformation has been laid. The art of Personal Alchemy invites us to see ourselves not as fixed entities but as ever-evolving beings, capable of profound change. It challenges us to look inward, to question, and to rebuild. Through the principles of NLP, we are offered tools to navigate this journey, to reshape our beliefs and behaviors with intention and creativity.

As the process begins, one cannot help but sense the magnitude of what lies ahead. Each step forward, no matter how small, is a step toward a life reimagined. The path of transformation is one of both discovery and creation, leading to a self that is not only new but also more authentically aligned with one's deepest truths.

Chapter 2
The Power of Now

The present moment is a paradox, fleeting yet eternal, elusive yet ever within reach. It is in this now, this sliver of time that defies definition, where the seeds of transformation are planted. To harness its power is to awaken to the reality that life does not unfold in the past we endlessly replay nor the future we ceaselessly project—it happens here, now, always.

But why is this so important for change? Because the now is where awareness lives. And awareness is the light that reveals the shadows of the mind, those automatic patterns that govern our thoughts, feelings, and actions. These patterns, entrenched by repetition, operate like invisible strings, puppeteering our responses without conscious consent. Breaking free from them requires stepping into the present, observing without judgment, and reclaiming choice.

To enter the now, however, is no simple task. The mind resists. It leaps to memories of yesterday or fears for tomorrow, seeking refuge in the familiarity of these realms. Here lies the first challenge: to quiet this ceaseless chatter and bring attention to what *is*. The breath becomes an anchor, grounding awareness in the body, in the rhythm of inhalation and exhalation. With each breath, the distractions recede, revealing a clarity untouched by the noise of time.

This practice is not merely a meditative exercise; it is the foundation of transformation. Awareness of the now exposes the mechanisms of the mind, those habitual thought loops and emotional reactions that perpetuate stagnation. Imagine a recurring frustration with a colleague. Without awareness, this frustration triggers the same response each time—an irritated comment, a sharp glance, a building resentment. But when presence illuminates this moment, a pause becomes possible. In that pause lies the freedom to choose differently, to respond instead of reacting.

Being present is not about perfection. Thoughts will drift, emotions will surge, and the mind will wander. The power lies in noticing when this happens and gently returning to the now. Over time, this return becomes a practice, a skill that strengthens like a muscle, offering ever greater insight into the inner workings of the self.

This insight is essential for transformation, for it uncovers the automatic programs running beneath awareness. These programs often originate in early experiences, where the mind, seeking to protect and adapt, created shortcuts. A child reprimanded for speaking too boldly may adopt a pattern of silence to avoid conflict. Decades later, as an adult, this same pattern persists, limiting the ability to assert oneself. Without awareness, the individual may never realize the origin of their behavior or that it no longer serves them.

Yet, the now offers more than just understanding. It provides a space to rewrite these programs. In the present moment, one can experiment with new ways of being—speaking up instead of staying silent, responding with kindness instead of defensiveness, choosing courage over fear. These small shifts, repeated and reinforced, begin to create new patterns that align with one's desires and values.

The challenge of remaining present becomes particularly evident in moments of discomfort. When faced with pain, whether physical, emotional, or psychological, the instinct is to flee—into distraction, denial, or numbing behaviors. But it is precisely in these moments that presence is most transformative. To stay, to feel, to breathe through the discomfort is to disarm its power. Pain, when met with awareness, loses its grip, revealing insights and lessons hidden beneath its surface.

One might ask: how does this practice of presence translate to the larger goals of transformation? The answer lies in its ability to disrupt the cycle of unconscious living. Every choice made in the now is a vote for the person one wishes to become. When one chooses presence over avoidance, authenticity over pretense, and intention over habit, they align with the process of change in its most organic form.

The present moment also serves as a mirror, reflecting the inner state with unflinching honesty. A restless mind, a tense body, a racing heart—all are signals, invitations to look deeper. What story is the mind telling? What belief is fueling this reaction? In this inquiry, guided by presence, one begins to peel back the layers of their conditioned responses, revealing the core beliefs and fears that drive them.

Yet, presence is not merely a tool for understanding the self. It is also the gateway to connection—with others, with the environment, and with the unfolding flow of life. A conversation held with full attention becomes a space for genuine exchange, free from the distractions of the past or future. A walk in nature, taken with presence, transforms into an immersion in the world's beauty and rhythm. Even mundane tasks, when approached with mindfulness, become opportunities for grounding and appreciation.

To fully embody the power of now is to recognize that transformation is not a distant goal but a continuous process happening in real time. It does not begin tomorrow, nor does it hinge on yesterday's failures. It begins in this breath, this moment, this choice. The journey of change unfolds step by step, with each present moment as a stepping stone.

As the practice of presence deepens, a profound shift occurs. The mind, once consumed by the noise of what was and what could be, begins to settle. A spaciousness emerges, a sense of being grounded in the here and now. In this space, creativity flourishes, intuition sharpens, and the possibilities for transformation expand.

The power of now is not just a concept but an experience, one that must be lived to be understood. It is the foundation upon which the entire journey of transformation rests, the compass that guides every step forward. To embrace it is to step into the fullness of life, where change is not a struggle but a natural unfolding, born of awareness and choice.

Chapter 3
Mapping the Mind

The human mind is a labyrinth, its pathways intricate and often obscured. To navigate it is to embark on a journey of self-discovery, one that reveals not only the mechanisms that drive thought and emotion but also the possibilities for profound transformation. Mapping the mind is the first step in this journey, an exploration that sheds light on the invisible patterns shaping perception, behavior, and identity.

Every individual carries within them a unique map of reality, a framework constructed from experiences, beliefs, and interpretations. This mental map is not a reflection of the world as it is but of the world as the individual perceives it. It filters every interaction, colors every memory, and guides every decision. To understand this map is to gain insight into the self and the forces that shape one's life.

This process begins with observation. Noticing thoughts as they arise, without judgment or attachment, is the foundation of self-awareness. The act of observing creates a separation between the thinker and the thought, allowing for a deeper understanding of how the mind operates. Patterns begin to emerge: recurring worries, automatic judgments, habitual reactions. These patterns are the pathways of the mental map, worn smooth by repetition.

Practical exercises can help illuminate these pathways. One such exercise involves tracking thoughts over a period of time, writing them down as they occur. This practice, often called a thought journal, reveals the themes and tendencies that dominate the mind. For instance, a person might notice a pattern of self-critical thoughts or a tendency to dwell on worst-case scenarios. Recognizing these patterns is the first step toward changing them.

Another technique is to pay attention to emotional responses. Emotions are powerful indicators of the mental map at work, often pointing to deeply held beliefs. A sudden surge of anger or fear, for example, may stem from an underlying belief about vulnerability or injustice. By tracing the emotion back to its source, one can uncover the belief driving it and begin to question its validity.

Understanding the concept of mental maps also involves recognizing their limitations. Every map is a simplification, a representation of reality rather than reality itself. The map is shaped by the individual's experiences, cultural background, and cognitive biases. It prioritizes some information while excluding or distorting other aspects. This is not a flaw but a necessary function of the mind, which cannot process the infinite complexity of the world. However, it becomes problematic when one mistakes the map for the territory, assuming their perspective is the only truth.

Expanding one's mental map requires a willingness to question assumptions and explore alternative perspectives. This process, often referred to as cognitive reframing, involves looking at situations through different lenses. For example, a failure might be reframed not as evidence of inadequacy but as an opportunity for growth. A conflict might be seen not as a threat but as a chance to build understanding. Each reframe adds depth and flexibility to the mental map.

The practice of mapping the mind also benefits from a focus on language. Words are the tools with which we construct our mental maps, shaping how we interpret and respond to the world. Consider the difference between saying, "I am bad at this," and, "I am learning this." The former statement reinforces a fixed, limiting belief, while the latter opens the door to growth. Becoming conscious of one's language patterns is a powerful way to reshape the mental map.

Visualization is another technique that aids in this process. By creating mental images of thoughts, emotions, or beliefs, one can make the abstract more tangible. For instance, a recurring fear might be visualized as a shadowy figure that follows at a distance. This image, once externalized, can be interacted with—shrunk, transformed, or confronted in a way that alters its influence. Visualization bridges the gap between the conscious and subconscious mind, making hidden patterns accessible.

Mapping the mind also involves recognizing its layers. The conscious mind, with its active thoughts and deliberate choices, is only the surface. Beneath it lies the subconscious, a vast reservoir of memories, beliefs, and instincts that exerts a profound influence on behavior. Accessing this deeper layer requires patience and subtlety. Techniques such as guided imagery, meditation, and NLP exercises can help uncover the subconscious patterns that shape the mental map.

A critical aspect of this exploration is the interplay between thoughts and emotions. They are not separate entities but deeply intertwined, each influencing the other in a continuous loop. A thought can trigger an emotional response, which in turn reinforces the thought. Breaking this loop requires disrupting the automatic connection between the two. For example, by challenging the thought, one can alter the emotional response it generates. Similarly, by calming the emotion—through breathing exercises, for instance—one can weaken the thought's grip.

As the mental map becomes clearer, its influence begins to shift. Awareness alone has a transformative power, allowing individuals to step outside their habitual patterns and choose new paths. This is the essence of personal transformation: not erasing the old map but expanding it, enriching it with new perspectives and possibilities.

The process of mapping the mind is ongoing, a dynamic practice rather than a one-time task. Just as the world around us changes, so too does the inner landscape. Staying attuned to these changes requires a commitment to self-reflection and growth. The map evolves as the individual evolves, becoming a truer and more flexible representation of their potential.

To map the mind is to embark on a journey of profound self-discovery. It is a practice of curiosity, courage, and creativity, one that unveils the intricate patterns of thought and emotion that shape our lives. In this exploration, the individual not only gains insight into their present state but also uncovers the tools to create their future. Every step taken in this process lays the groundwork for transformation, turning the once-mysterious labyrinth of the mind into a space of clarity, intention, and possibility.

Chapter 4
Limiting Beliefs

Deep within the recesses of the mind, unseen forces shape our lives. These forces, known as limiting beliefs, form the boundaries of what we perceive as possible. They are subtle yet pervasive, influencing decisions, actions, and even our sense of identity. To transform oneself is to confront these hidden constraints and reshape the narratives that hold us back.

Limiting beliefs begin as whispers, often rooted in early experiences. A child criticized for speaking out may grow into an adult who avoids sharing ideas, convinced their voice has little value. A single failure might spiral into a lifelong aversion to risk, fueled by the belief that success is unattainable. These beliefs are rarely questioned, accepted instead as truths that define the contours of reality.

Identifying limiting beliefs requires an unflinching look at the patterns of thought and behavior that dominate one's life. They often manifest as recurring themes: self-doubt, fear of failure, feelings of inadequacy. These patterns, while diverse in form, share a common thread—a narrative of restriction. To uncover them, one must ask probing questions: *What assumptions do I hold about myself? What do I believe I cannot do? What stories do I tell to justify staying within my comfort zone?*

The answers to these questions may not come easily. Limiting beliefs are elusive, cloaked in layers of rationalization and habit. Yet, certain phrases offer clues. Sentiments like "I'm not good enough," "I'll never succeed," or "That's just who I am" often signal the presence of a limiting belief. These statements, repeated over time, become self-fulfilling prophecies, shaping actions and outcomes in their image.

Once identified, the next step is to challenge these beliefs. This is no small task, for they are often deeply entrenched, woven into the fabric of one's identity. To challenge a belief is to question its validity: *Is this true? What evidence supports it? What evidence contradicts it?* Often, these inquiries reveal the fragility of the belief, exposing it as a construct rather than an immutable truth.

Consider a person who believes they are inherently bad at learning new skills. This belief may stem from a single experience—a failed attempt at mastering a complex task. Yet, when examined, it becomes clear that this isolated incident does not define their potential. By reframing the narrative—seeing failure not as a reflection of ability but as a natural part of the learning process—the belief begins to lose its hold.

Reframing is a powerful tool in dismantling limiting beliefs. It involves shifting perspective, finding alternative ways of interpreting experiences. For instance, instead of viewing rejection as a sign of inadequacy, one might see it as a step toward growth, an opportunity to refine and improve. This shift not only weakens the belief but also opens the door to new possibilities.

Language plays a critical role in this process. The words we use to describe ourselves and our circumstances can either reinforce limiting beliefs or pave the way for change. Phrases like "I can't" or "I'm not" trap us in a narrative of limitation. Replacing them with statements of possibility—"I can learn," "I'm improving"—creates a more empowering internal dialogue. These affirmations, though simple, have a profound impact on the subconscious, gradually reshaping self-perception.

Visualization is another technique that aids in overcoming limiting beliefs. By vividly imagining a version of oneself that embodies the desired qualities—confidence, resilience, creativity—one begins to bridge the gap between current reality and potential. The mind, unable to distinguish between real and vividly imagined experiences, integrates these visualizations as part of its narrative, reinforcing the belief in one's capacity for change.

Despite these tools, the process of confronting limiting beliefs is not without resistance. These beliefs often serve a protective function, shielding us from perceived threats. The fear of failure, for example, may discourage risk-taking, ostensibly safeguarding against disappointment. Yet, this protection comes at a cost, stifling growth and opportunity. Recognizing this dynamic is key to moving forward. It allows one to honor the belief's origins while choosing a new path.

Breaking free from limiting beliefs also requires patience. These narratives, formed over years or decades, will not dissolve overnight. Progress may be gradual, marked by small victories—choosing to speak up in a meeting, taking a chance on a new project, or simply acknowledging one's worth. Each step reinforces the new belief, creating a momentum that builds over time.

Support can be invaluable in this journey. Sharing one's experiences with trusted allies—friends, mentors, coaches—provides perspective and encouragement. Others often see strengths and possibilities that remain hidden from our own view, challenging the distorted lens of limiting beliefs. Their insights, combined with our own efforts, create a collaborative process of growth.

Ultimately, confronting limiting beliefs is an act of liberation. It is a reclaiming of power, a declaration that the stories of the past do not dictate the future. By dismantling these mental barriers, one creates space for new narratives, ones that reflect the vastness of human potential.

The journey does not end with the dissolution of a single belief. New challenges will arise, bringing fresh opportunities for introspection and growth. Each belief dismantled is a step closer to authenticity, to living a life not bound by fear but driven by possibility. To confront limiting beliefs is to embrace the fullness of one's humanity, to see not only the shadows but also the light within. And in this light, transformation becomes not just possible but inevitable.

22

Chapter 5
Reframing

Life is shaped not by events themselves but by the meanings we assign to them. Each moment, from the mundane to the profound, is filtered through the lens of perception, colored by personal experiences, beliefs, and emotions. This act of interpretation is both a gift and a limitation, for while it allows us to make sense of the world, it can also trap us in narratives that confine growth. The art of reframing offers a way out—a means to shift perspective and transform the meaning of experiences, unlocking new possibilities for thought and action.

Reframing begins with the recognition that meaning is not fixed. A single event can hold countless interpretations, each shaped by the viewer's mental framework. Consider a failure: one person might see it as evidence of inadequacy, while another views it as a stepping stone to success. The event itself remains unchanged, yet its impact differs profoundly based on the lens through which it is seen.

This understanding forms the foundation of reframing. To reframe is to consciously alter the lens, to choose a new narrative that empowers rather than limits. It is not about denying reality or avoiding discomfort but about finding perspectives that support growth and resilience. In this way, reframing becomes a tool for transformation, allowing individuals to rewrite their stories and reclaim agency over their lives.

The process of reframing begins with awareness. One must first identify the frames currently shaping their perception. These frames often operate unconsciously, embedded in habitual thoughts and language. A person who consistently says, "I'm unlucky," for instance, is framing their experiences through a lens of misfortune, filtering out evidence to the contrary. By becoming aware of such patterns, one can begin to question their validity.

Questioning is at the heart of reframing. It involves probing the assumptions underlying a given frame: *Is this interpretation the only possible one? What evidence supports it? What evidence challenges it? How might someone else view this situation?* These questions create mental space, opening the mind to alternative perspectives.

One powerful technique for reframing is shifting focus. This involves redirecting attention from the negative aspects of a situation to the positive or neutral ones. For example, losing a job might initially seem like a purely negative event. However, by shifting focus, one might see it as an opportunity to pursue a more fulfilling career or develop new skills. This shift does not erase the challenges involved but places them within a broader context that includes potential benefits.

Another approach is to reframe the meaning of challenges and setbacks. Rather than viewing obstacles as failures, one might see them as lessons, each providing valuable insights and experiences. This perspective transforms adversity into a catalyst for growth, fostering resilience and adaptability. It echoes the adage that life's greatest lessons often come from its greatest challenges.

Reframing can also be applied to relationships and interactions. Misunderstandings, conflicts, and criticisms are fertile ground for reframing, as they often involve entrenched narratives about oneself or others. For instance, receiving critical feedback might initially feel like a personal attack. By reframing, one might interpret the feedback as an opportunity to improve or as a sign that the other person values their potential. This shift not only reduces defensiveness but also creates space for constructive dialogue.

Language plays a central role in reframing, as the words we choose shape how we perceive and communicate experiences. Consider the difference between saying, "I have to do this," and,

"I get to do this." The former conveys obligation and resistance, while the latter emphasizes opportunity and choice. Such subtle shifts in phrasing can have a profound impact on mindset and motivation.

Visualization is another powerful tool for reframing. By imagining a situation from different angles, one can explore alternative interpretations and identify the most empowering frame. For instance, a person struggling with self-doubt might visualize themselves as a mentor offering guidance to a younger version of themselves. This exercise not only reframes their perspective but also taps into their inner wisdom and compassion.

Reframing is not always about finding a positive interpretation. Sometimes, it involves embracing complexity and nuance, recognizing that a situation can hold both pain and potential, loss and opportunity. This balanced perspective fosters acceptance and clarity, allowing one to navigate life's challenges with greater equanimity.

While reframing is a powerful practice, it requires effort and intention. The mind often resists change, clinging to familiar narratives even when they no longer serve. This resistance is rooted in the comfort of certainty, the desire to make sense of the world in predictable ways. Overcoming it requires persistence, as well as a willingness to confront the fears and insecurities underlying the current frame.

Support from others can also facilitate the reframing process. Trusted friends, mentors, or coaches can offer alternative perspectives, helping to challenge entrenched narratives and explore new possibilities. Their insights, combined with one's own reflections, create a collaborative process of transformation.

Ultimately, reframing is an act of empowerment. It reminds us that while we cannot always control what happens, we can control how we interpret and respond to it. This shift in perspective not only changes how we experience life but also influences the outcomes we create. By choosing frames that align with our values and aspirations, we take ownership of our stories, transforming them into vehicles of growth and fulfillment.

The practice of reframing is not a one-time effort but an ongoing journey. Life continually presents new challenges and opportunities, each offering a chance to explore and expand the frames through which we see the world. With each reframe, the mind becomes more flexible, the heart more open, and the self more aligned with its highest potential.

To reframe is to reclaim one's power—the power to shape meaning, to find purpose, and to create a life of intention and possibility. In this act, transformation becomes not just a destination but a way of being, a commitment to seeing the world not as it is but as it can be.

Chapter 6
Resource States

Deep within the human experience lies a reservoir of potential—moments of courage, joy, confidence, and calm that have shaped and guided us. These states, often fleeting, hold the power to transform how we approach challenges and opportunities. Resource states, as they are known, are the emotional and mental conditions that allow us to operate at our best. Learning to access, anchor, and amplify these states is a cornerstone of personal transformation.

Resource states are not foreign or unattainable. They are part of our lived experience, memories of times when we felt strong, capable, or resilient. A moment of pride after a hard-earned accomplishment, the calm focus during a creative flow, the unshakable confidence in the face of uncertainty—all these are resource states. The challenge is not in finding them but in making them readily available when needed.

The journey begins with identifying these states. This requires reflection, a search through memory for instances when you felt aligned with the qualities you now seek. Perhaps there was a time when you delivered a presentation with ease, even under pressure, or a moment when you comforted a friend and felt a deep sense of empathy. These memories, vivid and rich with emotion, are the key to unlocking resource states.

To harness the power of these states, one must first connect with their essence. Visualization is a powerful tool in this process. Close your eyes and recall a specific moment tied to the desired state. Engage your senses fully: What did you see? Hear? Feel? Immerse yourself in the memory until the emotion resurfaces, as if you are reliving it in the present. This connection strengthens the neural pathways associated with the state, making it more accessible over time.

Anchoring is a technique that takes this process a step further. It involves linking the resource state to a specific stimulus—a physical gesture, a word, or even a mental image—so that the state can be recalled on demand. For example, pressing your thumb and forefinger together while fully immersed in a memory of confidence creates an association between the gesture and the emotion. Repeating this practice reinforces the connection, allowing you to evoke confidence by simply performing the gesture in the future.

The choice of anchor is crucial. It should be distinct and easy to replicate in various situations. Physical gestures, such as clenching a fist or touching a specific part of the body, are particularly effective because they involve the sense of touch, which is deeply connected to memory. Verbal cues, like a phrase or mantra, can also serve as anchors, especially when paired with vivid visualization.

Once an anchor is established, it must be tested and strengthened. Begin by activating the anchor in a neutral or mildly challenging situation to ensure it triggers the desired state. With practice, the response will become automatic, providing a reliable tool to navigate moments of stress or uncertainty. Over time, multiple resource states can be anchored to different stimuli, creating a personalized toolkit for various scenarios.

Accessing resource states is not limited to individual experiences. Observing others who embody the qualities you seek can also serve as inspiration. This practice, often referred to as modeling, involves identifying role models and studying their behavior, language, and emotional demeanor. By mimicking these patterns, you can tap into similar resource states within yourself.

It's important to recognize that resource states are not static. They are dynamic, influenced by context, environment, and personal growth. A state that once felt empowering may evolve, giving way to new expressions of strength or confidence. Staying attuned to these changes ensures that your resource states remain relevant and effective.

Resource states also interact with one another, creating a synergy that enhances their impact. For example, combining the calm of mindfulness with the energy of motivation can result in focused determination, a state that balances intensity with clarity. Exploring these combinations deepens your understanding of emotional dynamics and expands your capacity to respond to complex situations.

Challenges will inevitably arise in this process. Stress, fatigue, or doubt can make resource states feel out of reach. In these moments, returning to the basics—breath, visualization, and anchoring—restores connection. Remember that the states themselves have not disappeared; they are simply waiting to be accessed with intention and patience.

The practice of accessing resource states is not confined to moments of need. It can also be integrated into daily routines to build resilience and enhance well-being. Morning rituals that involve recalling moments of gratitude or setting intentions for the day create a foundation of positivity and purpose. Similarly, evening reflections that focus on successes and lessons reinforce resourceful states for the future.

Ultimately, resource states are not just tools for specific challenges; they are pathways to a fuller, more empowered way of living. By cultivating these states, you align with the best version of yourself, drawing on inner strengths that are always present, even if momentarily obscured. They remind you that transformation is not about becoming something new but about reconnecting with what has always been within.

In mastering resource states, you create a bridge between potential and action. You gain the ability to meet life's complexities with grace, to find courage in vulnerability, and to act with clarity in the face of uncertainty. This mastery is not an endpoint but a continuous process of discovery, an ongoing dance with the ever-changing rhythms of the self.

As resource states become second nature, they transform from fleeting moments into enduring qualities. Confidence, resilience, and calm become not just states but traits, integral to who you are and how you move through the world. Through this practice, you step into your power, equipped not only to navigate life's challenges but to embrace its infinite possibilities.

Chapter 7
Identifying Patterns

Human behavior is a tapestry woven from recurring threads—patterns of thought, emotion, and action that shape our lives. These patterns, though often invisible to the untrained eye, are the scripts that dictate how we respond to the world. They are the habits we repeat, the triggers that ignite us, and the cycles we find ourselves caught in, time and again. Identifying these patterns is a crucial step in the journey of transformation, for what is observed can be understood, and what is understood can be changed.

Patterns originate in the mind's natural tendency to seek efficiency. Faced with the overwhelming complexity of life, the brain simplifies, creating shortcuts for navigating familiar situations. These shortcuts, known as heuristics, are often useful, conserving mental energy and enabling quick decision-making. However, when left unchecked, they can solidify into rigid patterns that limit flexibility and growth.

To uncover these patterns, one must cultivate a mindset of curiosity and observation. This begins with self-awareness, a deliberate focus on the interplay of thoughts, emotions, and behaviors in everyday life. Like a detective examining clues, the individual learns to notice the recurring themes and triggers that influence their actions.

Triggers are among the most revealing aspects of patterns. They are the stimuli—internal or external—that spark a specific response. A harsh comment from a colleague might trigger defensiveness, or a looming deadline might ignite anxiety. Identifying these triggers requires attentiveness, a willingness to pause in the moment and ask, *What just happened? What am I reacting to?* Over time, this practice reveals the chain of events that connects trigger to response.

Journaling is a powerful tool for capturing and analyzing patterns. By recording thoughts, feelings, and actions throughout the day, one can create a map of their inner world. Patterns that might go unnoticed in the moment become clear when reviewed over time. For instance, a journal might reveal that feelings of frustration consistently arise after interactions with a specific individual or in response to certain tasks. This awareness transforms the pattern from an unconscious loop into a solvable puzzle.

Another effective technique is mindfulness. By cultivating a nonjudgmental awareness of the present moment, mindfulness allows one to observe patterns as they unfold. Imagine feeling a surge of anger during a conversation. Instead of reacting impulsively, mindfulness creates space to notice the anger, explore its origins, and choose a measured response. This practice not only interrupts unhelpful patterns but also builds the capacity for intentionality.

Recognizing emotional patterns is especially important, as emotions are powerful drivers of behavior. Emotional triggers often stem from unmet needs or unresolved experiences, surfacing as recurring reactions. For example, a pattern of withdrawing during conflict might point to a deep-seated fear of rejection, while a tendency to overcommit might reflect a need for approval. Exploring these connections requires honesty and compassion, a willingness to confront uncomfortable truths without self-judgment.

Behavioral patterns are equally significant. Habits, routines, and automatic responses form the structure of daily life, shaping outcomes in ways both subtle and profound. Some patterns, like exercising regularly or practicing gratitude, support well-being and growth. Others, like procrastination or negative self-talk, create obstacles. Identifying which patterns serve and which hinder is a key step in the transformation process.

The body, too, holds patterns, often reflecting emotional and mental states. Posture, gestures, and tension reveal insights that words cannot. A clenched jaw might indicate suppressed anger, while slouched shoulders signal resignation or low confidence. By paying attention to these physical cues, one gains a deeper understanding of the interplay between mind and body.

Relationships are another rich source of patterns. Interactions with others often follow predictable scripts, shaped by individual dynamics and shared histories. Perhaps there is a pattern of conflict with a particular family member or a tendency to avoid difficult conversations with a partner. These relational patterns, while challenging to confront, hold immense potential for growth. By recognizing them, one can begin to shift the dynamics and create healthier connections.

Breaking unhelpful patterns requires both insight and action. Insight comes from observing and understanding the pattern—its triggers, its consequences, and the beliefs that sustain it. Action involves experimenting with new responses, testing alternative ways of thinking and behaving. For instance, instead of reacting defensively to criticism, one might practice active listening, seeking to understand the other person's perspective. This shift not only disrupts the pattern but also fosters personal growth and improved relationships.

It is important to approach this process with patience. Patterns are often deeply ingrained, built over years or even decades. Changing them is not a matter of willpower alone but of persistence and self-compassion. Setbacks are inevitable, but each attempt to shift a pattern contributes to the larger goal of transformation.

Support from others can be invaluable in this journey. Friends, mentors, or therapists provide perspective and encouragement, helping to illuminate patterns that may be difficult to see on one's own. Their insights, combined with personal reflection, create a more comprehensive understanding of the patterns at play.

As new patterns take root, they create a ripple effect, transforming not only the individual but also their environment. A shift in mindset or behavior often inspires similar changes in those around them, fostering a culture of growth and resilience. Over time, the cumulative impact of these changes reshapes the individual's experience of life, aligning it more closely with their values and aspirations.

The process of identifying and shifting patterns is an ongoing one. Life continually presents new challenges and opportunities, each revealing fresh layers of the self. With each cycle of observation and change, the individual becomes more adept at navigating the complexities of their inner world, turning patterns of limitation into pathways of possibility.

Ultimately, identifying patterns is an act of liberation. It frees the individual from the constraints of unconscious habits, enabling them to live with greater awareness, intention, and authenticity. In this freedom, transformation becomes not a distant goal but a lived reality, unfolding moment by moment, pattern by pattern.

Chapter 8
Transformative Language

Words are not merely tools for communication; they are the architects of reality. The language we use, both spoken and unspoken, has the power to shape our thoughts, influence our emotions, and define our actions. Transformative language harnesses this power, offering a pathway to reframe experiences, challenge limitations, and inspire change. To master this art is to unlock a profound tool for personal growth and self-transformation.

Language operates on two levels. The external, or spoken, language shapes how we communicate with others, influencing relationships and interactions. The internal, or self-directed, language governs the ongoing narrative within our minds. Both levels are deeply interconnected, each reinforcing the other in a continuous cycle of meaning and interpretation.

The journey toward transformative language begins with awareness. What words do you habitually use to describe yourself, your circumstances, and the world around you? These words often reveal underlying beliefs and attitudes, offering a window into the mental and emotional patterns driving behavior. For example, describing oneself as "overwhelmed" or "stuck" reinforces a narrative of helplessness, while framing a challenge as an "opportunity to grow" creates a foundation for empowerment.

One technique for cultivating awareness is journaling. Writing down thoughts as they arise helps capture the language of the mind, providing a tangible record for reflection. Patterns often emerge in this process—phrases that recur, themes that dominate.

These patterns are the raw material for transformation, highlighting areas where language can be reshaped to support growth.

Reframing is central to transformative language. It involves consciously replacing disempowering words and phrases with ones that align with a desired mindset. Consider the difference between saying, "I failed," and, "I learned something valuable." The first statement shuts down possibilities, while the second opens the door to reflection and growth. Reframing does not deny reality but rather interprets it through a lens that fosters resilience and progress.

Affirmations are another powerful tool for transformation. These are positive, present-tense statements that reinforce desired beliefs and behaviors. For example, "I am capable of overcoming challenges" or "I deserve success and happiness." Repeating affirmations daily, whether aloud or in writing, helps embed them into the subconscious, gradually replacing limiting narratives with empowering ones.

The structure of language also plays a crucial role. Subtle shifts in phrasing can create significant changes in perception. Compare the statements, "I have to do this" and "I get to do this." The former implies obligation and resistance, while the latter emphasizes opportunity and gratitude. Similarly, replacing "but" with "and" encourages inclusivity rather than conflict: "I want to rest, and I also want to finish this task."

Metaphors and imagery are particularly effective in transformative language, as they engage the subconscious mind directly. Describing a journey of change as "planting seeds and watching them grow" evokes patience, nurturing, and potential. A metaphor like "breaking through a wall" conveys determination and progress. By choosing metaphors that resonate personally, one can create a vivid mental framework that supports transformation.

Body language, though often overlooked, is an essential part of this process. The way we hold ourselves—posture, gestures, facial expressions—communicates powerful messages to both the self and others. Standing tall, maintaining open gestures, and smiling can reinforce feelings of confidence and approachability. Conversely, slouched postures or closed-off gestures often mirror and perpetuate states of insecurity or defensiveness. Becoming conscious of this physical dimension adds depth to the practice of transformative language.

Transformative language also extends to interactions with others. How we speak to those around us reflects and reinforces our internal state. Encouraging, empathetic language not only strengthens relationships but also fosters a supportive inner dialogue. Conversely, critical or dismissive language can create tension and mirror self-criticism. Practicing mindful communication—choosing words with care, listening actively, and expressing thoughts with clarity—enhances both external and internal harmony.

Challenging conversations offer a unique opportunity to practice transformative language. Instead of reacting defensively or aggressively, one can choose words that de-escalate conflict and promote understanding. For example, expressing needs through "I" statements—such as "I feel unheard when..." rather than "You never listen"—shifts the focus from blame to resolution. This approach not only diffuses tension but also models constructive communication for others.

The subconscious mind plays a pivotal role in shaping behavior, and language is its primary interface. Hypnotic language patterns, such as those used in Neuro-Linguistic Programming (NLP), tap into this subconscious realm to create change. These patterns include the use of positive suggestions, embedded commands, and open-ended questions that guide the mind toward desired outcomes. For instance, asking, "What new possibilities might arise if I embrace this challenge?" directs attention to opportunities rather than obstacles.

While transformative language is a powerful tool, its practice requires consistency and intention. Old patterns of speech, deeply ingrained through habit, will not dissolve overnight. It takes time to replace them with new, empowering alternatives. Each choice of words, each reframed thought, builds momentum, gradually rewiring the mind for growth and resilience.

Feedback from others can be invaluable in this process. Friends, mentors, or coaches can reflect back the language you use, offering insights into unconscious patterns and suggesting alternatives. Their perspective helps illuminate blind spots, accelerating the journey toward mastery.

The impact of transformative language extends far beyond the individual. As one's internal dialogue shifts, so too does their external presence. Relationships become more authentic, interactions more meaningful, and communication more impactful. This ripple effect fosters an environment of growth and positivity, influencing not only the self but also those around.

Ultimately, transformative language is more than a tool; it is a way of being. It reflects a commitment to conscious living, to choosing words that align with one's highest values and aspirations. Through this practice, the individual becomes both author and editor of their story, crafting a narrative that inspires and uplifts.

In mastering the art of transformative language, one discovers the profound truth that words are not just reflections of thought—they are instruments of creation. With every phrase, every sentence, we shape the contours of our reality, forging paths toward the life we seek to live. Through this practice, transformation becomes not just a possibility but a certainty, written in the language of intention and possibility.

Chapter 9
The Inner Mirror

There is a mirror within each of us, one that reflects not our outward appearance but the depths of our inner world. This mirror holds the truths of who we are—our strengths, fears, aspirations, and limitations. Yet, it is often clouded by judgment, distorted by criticism, and obscured by the weight of expectation. The practice of gazing into this inner mirror with clarity and compassion is a transformative act, one that fosters self-acceptance and unlocks the path to growth.

Self-acceptance begins with the courage to observe without judgment. The mind, conditioned by societal norms and personal experiences, tends to evaluate every thought, feeling, and action through a critical lens. This inner critic often speaks in harsh tones, magnifying perceived flaws and dismissing accomplishments. To quiet this voice, one must first recognize its presence, bringing awareness to the narrative it perpetuates.

The practice of non-judgmental observation is a cornerstone of this process. It involves stepping back from the stream of thoughts and emotions, viewing them as an impartial witness. Instead of labeling a mistake as "failure" or a feeling of sadness as "weakness," one simply acknowledges their existence: *I made an error. I feel sadness.* This shift from judgment to observation creates space for understanding and growth.

A powerful tool in this journey is self-inquiry. By asking reflective questions, one can uncover the deeper layers of the inner mirror. *What am I feeling right now? Why does this situation trigger me? What belief lies beneath this reaction?* These questions, approached with curiosity rather than judgment, reveal the patterns and stories shaping one's inner world. Over time, this practice illuminates not only the surface reflections but also the underlying truths.

Compassion is the balm that clears the mirror. To meet oneself with kindness, especially in moments of struggle, is to cultivate a relationship of trust and acceptance with the self. This does not mean excusing harmful behaviors or ignoring areas for improvement but rather approaching them with understanding. A mistake, when viewed with compassion, becomes an opportunity to learn rather than a source of shame.

One technique for fostering self-compassion is the practice of self-affirmation. This involves consciously affirming one's worth and humanity, even in the face of imperfection. Phrases like *I am doing my best, I am enough as I am,* or *I deserve kindness* serve as reminders that flaws do not diminish value. These affirmations, repeated regularly, help reframe the inner dialogue, replacing criticism with encouragement.

The inner mirror also reflects our relationship with emotions. Many people, conditioned to view certain emotions as "negative" or "undesirable," suppress or avoid feelings like anger, sadness, or fear. However, these emotions are not enemies but messengers, signaling unmet needs or unresolved issues. By allowing these feelings to surface and exploring their origins, one can transform them from sources of pain into catalysts for growth.

Visualization can aid in this process. Imagine the inner mirror as a literal object, perhaps fogged or cracked, and visualize clearing it. Each act of self-reflection, each moment of compassion, becomes a gesture of polishing the glass, revealing a truer image. This exercise not only reinforces the practice of self-acceptance but also creates a tangible representation of the inner work being done.

The role of the body in this practice is equally important. Physical sensations often provide clues to the emotions and thoughts reflected in the inner mirror. A tight chest might signal anxiety, while a relaxed posture reflects ease. By tuning into these sensations, one gains a deeper connection to their inner state, bridging the gap between mind and body.

Relationships serve as external mirrors, reflecting aspects of the self that may be difficult to see alone. The dynamics of interactions often reveal hidden beliefs and patterns. For instance, a tendency to avoid conflict might reflect a fear of rejection, while repeated frustrations with others might point to unmet personal expectations. By examining these reflections, one gains insight into how their inner world shapes their external experiences.

While the inner mirror offers profound opportunities for growth, it also demands honesty. To see oneself clearly is to confront not only strengths but also weaknesses, not only achievements but also regrets. This honesty, though uncomfortable, is essential for transformation. It allows one to accept the full spectrum of their humanity, embracing both light and shadow.

The act of acceptance does not mean resignation. Accepting oneself as they are in the present moment is not the same as abandoning the desire for growth. On the contrary, self-acceptance creates a stable foundation for change, freeing the individual from the burden of self-rejection. From this place of acceptance, transformation becomes a choice made from love rather than fear.

Over time, the practice of gazing into the inner mirror reveals a deeper truth: the self is not a fixed entity but an evolving process. Each reflection, each insight, contributes to the ongoing story of who we are becoming. This understanding fosters a sense of curiosity and openness, encouraging one to approach life as an exploration rather than a test.

The clarity gained from this practice extends beyond the self. As the inner mirror becomes clearer, it enhances the ability to connect authentically with others. By accepting oneself, one becomes more accepting of others, creating relationships rooted in empathy and understanding. This ripple effect transforms not only the individual but also their environment, fostering a culture of growth and compassion.

To look into the inner mirror is to embark on a journey of self-discovery, one that requires courage, patience, and commitment. It is a practice of seeing oneself fully and loving what is seen, not in spite of imperfections but because of them. Through this act of reflection, the individual steps into their power, embracing the beauty and complexity of their humanity.

The inner mirror is both a guide and a companion on the path of transformation. It reminds us that the answers we seek are not found in the external world but within, waiting to be uncovered. In its reflection, we find not only who we are but also who we can become, illuminated by the light of self-acceptance and the infinite potential for growth.

Chapter 10
Creative Visualization

The mind is a canvas, vast and boundless, upon which the imagination paints the visions of what could be. Creative visualization harnesses this innate power, transforming abstract dreams into tangible realities. It is the art of shaping the unseen into the seen, aligning thoughts and emotions with intention to manifest change. This practice is not merely a tool for goal-setting but a profound gateway to transformation, connecting the conscious and subconscious in a dance of possibility.

At its core, creative visualization relies on the principle that the mind does not distinguish between vividly imagined experiences and reality. When we visualize an event or outcome with clarity and emotion, the brain responds as though it is already happening. This process strengthens neural pathways, primes the subconscious for action, and fosters a sense of belief that propels us toward our goals.

The practice begins with clarity of intention. What is it that you seek to create or achieve? A vague desire—"I want to be happy" or "I want success"—lacks the focus needed to engage the mind fully. Instead, define your intention with precision. If happiness is the goal, ask yourself: *What does happiness look like for me? What specific experiences, relationships, or states of being contribute to this feeling?* This specificity transforms an abstract idea into a clear vision.

Once the intention is set, the process of visualization unfolds in layers. Find a quiet space where you can focus without distraction. Close your eyes and bring the desired outcome to life in your mind. Engage all your senses to make the image as vivid as possible. What do you see? Hear? Feel? Smell? Even taste? The more detail you include, the more real the visualization becomes, activating the brain's full spectrum of sensory processing.

Emotion is the fuel that drives this process. Visualizing an outcome in a detached or mechanical way limits its effectiveness. Instead, immerse yourself in the feelings associated with the vision. If you are visualizing a professional achievement, feel the pride, joy, and excitement of success. If you are envisioning a personal goal, such as improved relationships, allow yourself to experience the warmth, connection, and love that accompany it. These emotions create a powerful resonance between your inner state and the desired reality.

Repetition reinforces the neural connections formed during visualization. Make it a daily practice, dedicating time each morning or evening to focus on your vision. Like water carving a path through stone, repeated visualization deepens the imprint on the subconscious, making the desired outcome feel not only possible but inevitable.

While visualization is a practice of the mind, its effects extend into action. The images and emotions cultivated during this process inspire choices and behaviors that align with the vision. A person who visualizes themselves as confident and capable is more likely to take risks, pursue opportunities, and embody those qualities in daily life. The mind and body work in harmony, translating thought into movement.

Visualization can also be used to overcome obstacles and challenges. When faced with fear or doubt, visualize yourself navigating the situation successfully. See yourself meeting adversity with resilience, finding solutions, and emerging stronger. This mental rehearsal not only reduces anxiety but also prepares you to respond effectively when the moment arises.

The practice of creative visualization is not limited to future outcomes; it can also be applied to healing and self-discovery. Visualizing the release of tension, the mending of emotional wounds, or the activation of inner strength fosters a sense of wholeness and empowerment. These internal transformations ripple outward, influencing how you engage with the world.

Vision boards offer a tangible extension of creative visualization. By assembling images, words, and symbols that represent your goals and aspirations, you create a physical reminder of your vision. Placing the board where it is seen daily reinforces the connection between your conscious and subconscious mind, keeping your goals at the forefront of your awareness.

Despite its power, visualization is not a substitute for action. It is a complement, a preparatory step that aligns the mind and spirit with the path ahead. Goals are realized through the synergy of thought and effort, intention and movement. Visualization provides the mental blueprint, but it is the actions you take that bring the vision to life.

Doubt and skepticism may arise during this process, particularly if the goal feels distant or unattainable. Address these feelings with curiosity rather than resistance. Ask yourself: *What beliefs are creating this doubt? How can I reframe them to support my vision?* Acknowledge the skepticism, but do not let it dominate. Return to the visualization with renewed focus and faith in your ability to create change.

Collaboration can enhance the power of visualization. Sharing your vision with supportive individuals fosters accountability and encouragement. Group visualization practices, where collective energy amplifies the impact, can also be a profound experience, uniting shared intentions in a dynamic field of possibility.

Over time, the practice of creative visualization reshapes not only the outcomes you pursue but also the way you perceive yourself and the world. It cultivates a mindset of abundance and opportunity, shifting focus from limitations to possibilities. The act of envisioning a better future becomes a declaration of agency, a reminder that you are not merely a spectator in life but an active creator.

The beauty of creative visualization lies in its adaptability. Whether used to achieve specific goals, navigate challenges, or deepen self-awareness, it is a practice that evolves with you. Each vision, each intention, becomes a stepping stone in the continuous journey of transformation.

Through this practice, the boundaries between imagination and reality blur, revealing the profound truth that the life you envision is within reach. It begins not in the external world but in the quiet space of the mind, where creativity and intention converge. In this space, transformation takes root, growing steadily until the imagined becomes real, and the vision becomes life itself.

Chapter 11
Conscious Communication

Communication is the bridge that connects thoughts to action, emotions to understanding, and individuals to one another. At its most basic, it is the transfer of information; at its most profound, it is the vehicle for transformation. Conscious communication is the practice of bringing awareness and intention to every interaction—both with others and within oneself. It requires clarity, empathy, and authenticity, creating a foundation for meaningful connections and personal growth.

The journey toward conscious communication begins with self-awareness. Every conversation, whether external or internal, is shaped by underlying thoughts, emotions, and assumptions. These often operate below the level of consciousness, influencing tone, word choice, and interpretation. By becoming aware of these influences, one gains the ability to choose responses that align with their values and goals, rather than reacting automatically.

Listening is the cornerstone of conscious communication. True listening goes beyond hearing words; it involves fully attending to the speaker, seeking to understand their perspective without judgment or interruption. This level of presence requires patience and a willingness to set aside one's own agenda. Active listening techniques—such as maintaining eye contact, nodding in acknowledgment, and paraphrasing the speaker's message—demonstrate respect and foster trust.

Empathy deepens this connection, enabling one to tune into the emotions and experiences behind the words. It is not about agreeing with the other person but about validating their feelings and showing that their perspective matters. Simple statements like *"That sounds challenging"* or *"I can see why you feel that way"* convey empathy and encourage open dialogue. This creates a safe space for honest communication, where both parties feel seen and heard.

The role of language in conscious communication cannot be overstated. Words have the power to build bridges or erect barriers, to heal or to harm. Choosing words with care, especially in emotionally charged situations, is a hallmark of conscious communication. For instance, replacing accusatory statements like *"You always ignore me"* with *"I feel unheard when..."* shifts the focus from blame to resolution. This approach invites collaboration rather than defensiveness, paving the way for constructive outcomes.

Nonverbal communication adds another layer of complexity and richness. Facial expressions, gestures, posture, and tone of voice all convey meaning, often more powerfully than words. A calm tone and open posture signal approachability, while crossed arms and a furrowed brow may indicate defensiveness or disinterest. Becoming attuned to these cues in oneself and others enhances understanding and helps align verbal and nonverbal messages for greater authenticity.

Clarity is essential in conscious communication. Ambiguity or vagueness can lead to misunderstandings, frustration, and conflict. To communicate clearly, one must articulate thoughts and feelings with precision, avoiding assumptions or expectations that others should "just know." This includes stating needs, boundaries, and intentions explicitly. For example, instead of saying, *"You never help,"* specify the desired action: *"It would mean a lot if you could assist me with this task."*

Internal communication is equally critical, as the way we speak to ourselves shapes our mindset and actions. Negative self-talk—*"I always mess things up"* or *"I'm not good enough"*—creates a narrative of limitation and doubt. Replacing these statements with affirming language—*"I am learning and growing"* or *"I am capable of handling challenges"*—fosters a more supportive and empowering inner dialogue.

Conflict provides a unique opportunity for practicing conscious communication. Disagreements often arise from unmet needs, misaligned expectations, or misunderstandings. Approaching conflict with a mindset of curiosity rather than combativeness transforms it into a chance for growth. Asking open-ended questions—*"Can you help me understand your perspective?"*—and expressing one's own needs without blame—*"I feel frustrated because..."*—facilitates resolution and strengthens relationships.

Conscious communication also requires awareness of power dynamics and cultural contexts. Words and actions carry different meanings depending on the relationships and backgrounds of those involved. Sensitivity to these nuances fosters inclusivity and respect, ensuring that communication uplifts rather than marginalizes.

One of the most powerful tools in conscious communication is the pause. In moments of tension or emotion, pausing before responding allows time to process and choose words thoughtfully. This practice helps prevent impulsive reactions and ensures that the response aligns with one's intentions.

Practicing conscious communication does not mean avoiding mistakes. Misunderstandings and missteps are inevitable, even with the best intentions. The key is to acknowledge them openly, apologize when necessary, and seek to repair the connection. This humility and willingness to learn strengthens relationships and builds trust.

Over time, conscious communication becomes more than a skill; it becomes a way of being. It fosters authenticity, where words and actions reflect one's true self. It nurtures relationships, creating bonds built on trust and understanding. And it enhances self-awareness, deepening the connection between thoughts, feelings, and actions.

In mastering conscious communication, one discovers its transformative potential. It is not merely about exchanging information but about creating meaningful connections—connections that inspire growth, foster empathy, and align with the deepest truths of who we are. Through this practice, communication becomes a bridge to transformation, both within and beyond ourselves.

Chapter 12
The Power of Empathy

Empathy is the quiet force that bridges the gap between individuals, fostering connection, understanding, and trust. It is more than an emotion; it is a skill, a choice, and a practice that transforms relationships and deepens the human experience. In the journey of personal transformation, empathy serves as both a mirror and a window—a reflection of one's own growth and a view into the hearts of others.

At its essence, empathy is the ability to sense, understand, and share the feelings of another. It is not about fixing, solving, or advising but about being present, offering a safe space for someone to express themselves fully. This presence creates a profound sense of being seen and valued, a cornerstone of authentic connection.

Empathy begins with listening—not just hearing words but attuning to the emotions and intentions behind them. This requires setting aside distractions and judgments, tuning in with full attention. Active listening techniques, such as paraphrasing what the other person has said or reflecting their feelings, demonstrate understanding. Phrases like *"It sounds like you're feeling..."* or *"I hear that this is really important to you"* validate their experience and encourage openness.

Yet empathy extends beyond verbal communication. It involves reading nonverbal cues—facial expressions, body language, tone of voice—that often convey more than words alone. A trembling voice may reveal fear; averted eyes might suggest discomfort. By observing these signals with care, one gains deeper insight into the emotions being expressed.

Empathy is not limited to understanding others; it also involves self-awareness. Recognizing one's own emotions and biases is essential to avoid projecting them onto others. For instance, feeling anxious about a situation might color how one interprets another person's actions, leading to misunderstandings. Practicing mindfulness and reflection helps separate personal feelings from the emotions of those around us, ensuring that empathy remains clear and genuine.

Cultivating empathy also requires humility—the acknowledgment that one cannot fully know another's experience. Even with the best intentions, assumptions and judgments can cloud understanding. Asking open-ended questions, such as *"Can you tell me more about what this feels like for you?"* invites the other person to share their perspective without interference. This openness fosters a sense of mutual respect and collaboration.

One of the most transformative aspects of empathy is its ability to reveal common ground. While individual experiences are unique, the emotions underlying them—joy, sorrow, fear, love—are universal. Recognizing these shared feelings creates a sense of connection that transcends differences. It reminds us that, at our core, we are all human, navigating the complexities of life in our own ways.

Empathy also plays a pivotal role in conflict resolution. Disagreements often stem from unacknowledged emotions or unmet needs. By approaching conflict with empathy, one can move beyond the surface issues to address the deeper concerns. For example, instead of arguing over specific actions, one might explore the feelings driving those actions: *"I see that you're upset. Can you help me understand what's behind that?"* This shift from confrontation to curiosity paves the way for understanding and resolution.

In addition to transforming relationships, empathy is a powerful tool for personal growth. The act of understanding others often mirrors back insights about oneself. Observing someone else's courage, for instance, might inspire similar strength within. Conversely, recognizing the impact of one's actions on others can highlight areas for improvement. Empathy thus becomes a catalyst for self-awareness and transformation.

Empathy is not without its challenges. It requires emotional energy and can sometimes lead to feelings of overwhelm, particularly when engaging with others' pain or suffering. To sustain empathy without depleting oneself, it is important to practice boundaries and self-care. This does not mean closing off but rather balancing compassion for others with compassion for oneself. Techniques such as deep breathing, mindfulness, and time for reflection help maintain this balance.

Compassionate detachment is another key aspect of sustainable empathy. This involves offering understanding and support without taking on responsibility for another's emotions or choices. It allows one to remain present and caring while recognizing that each individual must navigate their own path.

Empathy is also a tool for broader societal transformation. By fostering understanding and connection, it bridges divides and promotes inclusivity. In a world often fractured by conflict and misunderstanding, empathy has the power to heal and unite. Practicing empathy in everyday interactions—whether with colleagues, strangers, or loved ones—contributes to a culture of respect and kindness that ripples outward.

The practice of empathy is both a skill and a mindset. It deepens with intention and effort, becoming a natural part of how one engages with the world. Over time, it reshapes not only relationships but also the way one views life itself, fostering a sense of interconnectedness and shared humanity.

Empathy, ultimately, is a reflection of growth. It reveals the capacity to move beyond the self, to embrace the complexity and beauty of others' experiences. In its practice, one discovers the profound truth that transformation is not an individual journey but a shared one, enriched by the connections we nurture along the way.

Chapter 13
Positive Anchors

Within the tapestry of human experience, certain moments stand out—instances of joy, confidence, serenity, or triumph. These moments, rich with emotion and meaning, often feel fleeting, slipping through the grasp of memory as time marches on. Yet, these experiences hold immense transformative potential. Positive anchoring, a technique rooted in Neuro-Linguistic Programming (NLP), offers a method to capture and harness these moments, creating reliable triggers for desired emotional states.

Anchors are stimuli—physical, visual, auditory, or otherwise—that become associated with a specific emotional or mental state. They are akin to bookmarks in the mind, allowing us to return to the exact feeling of a past moment with intentional precision. For instance, a particular song might evoke nostalgia for a cherished time, or the scent of a favorite dish might bring comfort and warmth. Positive anchors deliberately create these associations, enabling access to empowering states when needed.

The practice begins with identifying moments that embody the desired state. Reflect on instances where you felt truly alive, confident, peaceful, or capable. These moments need not be grand; even simple experiences, such as a heartfelt laugh with a friend or the quiet satisfaction of completing a task, can serve as anchors. The key is the intensity and authenticity of the emotion felt during the experience.

Once a moment is selected, the next step is to vividly relive it. Close your eyes and immerse yourself in the memory. Engage all your senses: *What did you see? What sounds surrounded you? What textures, scents, or tastes were present?* Allow the emotions to rise, as if the memory is happening in the present. The more vividly the memory is re-experienced, the stronger the anchor will be.

While fully immersed in the emotion, introduce a unique and repeatable stimulus. This might be a physical gesture, such as pressing your thumb and forefinger together, a specific word or phrase, or even a deep breath in a particular pattern. The stimulus should be simple and easy to replicate, ensuring it can be used consistently. By pairing this stimulus with the peak of the emotional experience, the association between the two becomes encoded in the mind.

Repetition strengthens the anchor. Over time, revisiting the memory and pairing it with the stimulus reinforces the connection, making it increasingly automatic. With practice, activating the stimulus alone will elicit the desired state, even in challenging situations. For example, pressing your thumb and forefinger together might instantly evoke calm during a stressful meeting or confidence before a presentation.

Anchors are not limited to past experiences; they can also be created from imagined scenarios. Visualization, a powerful tool in its own right, allows you to construct vivid, positive states even if you have not yet experienced them in reality. By imagining yourself achieving a goal, feeling empowered, or thriving in a new environment, and pairing this visualization with a stimulus, you create an anchor for future possibilities.

The versatility of positive anchoring extends beyond individual emotions to more complex states of being. Combining multiple anchors can create a layered effect, addressing a variety of needs. For instance, a combination of calm and focus might be anchored for use during high-pressure tasks, while confidence and compassion could be paired for navigating difficult conversations. This flexibility allows you to tailor anchors to specific contexts and goals.

While positive anchoring is a powerful technique, its effectiveness relies on regular practice and mindful application. Anchors can fade over time if not revisited, so it is essential to refresh them periodically by revisiting the original memory or visualization. This upkeep ensures that the emotional connection remains strong and accessible.

It is also important to be aware of unintentional anchors. Just as positive states can be deliberately anchored, negative states can become inadvertently tied to stimuli through repeated association. For instance, a particular tone of voice or environment might trigger feelings of anxiety or frustration. Recognizing these patterns allows you to disrupt and replace them with intentional positive anchors, breaking cycles of unhelpful responses.

Anchors can be incorporated into daily routines, creating moments of alignment and grounding. A deep breath taken with a deliberate anchor might start the day with clarity, while a brief gesture paired with a positive state can reset focus during a busy afternoon. These practices transform anchoring into a seamless part of life, weaving empowerment into the fabric of everyday experiences.

Beyond personal growth, anchoring can enhance interactions with others. Sharing or introducing positive stimuli in relationships—such as a shared phrase, gesture, or ritual—creates connections rooted in uplifting emotions. These shared anchors not only strengthen bonds but also foster mutual support in moments of challenge.

As with any transformative practice, anchoring requires patience and experimentation. Not every anchor will resonate equally, and some may require refinement to achieve the desired effect. Embrace this process as a journey of discovery, one that deepens your understanding of your own emotional landscape.

Ultimately, positive anchors serve as a bridge between intention and action, thought and emotion. They provide a means to access your best self, even in the midst of uncertainty or adversity. By consciously creating and utilizing these anchors, you reclaim agency over your emotional states, empowering yourself to navigate life's complexities with resilience and grace.

In mastering the art of positive anchoring, you unlock a profound resource within—a reservoir of strength, joy, and confidence that is always accessible. Through this practice, the moments that once felt fleeting become lasting sources of empowerment, transforming not only how you feel but also how you live, connect, and create.

Chapter 14
State Breaking

Human behavior is guided by patterns, automatic responses deeply ingrained through repetition and experience. While these patterns often serve a purpose—streamlining decisions, conserving energy—they can also confine, creating rigid loops that limit growth and adaptability. State breaking is the practice of disrupting these patterns, offering a way to interrupt automatic behaviors and create space for intentional change. It is a tool for liberation, allowing individuals to step out of old cycles and into new possibilities.

A state, in the context of personal transformation, refers to the combination of emotions, thoughts, and physical sensations that define how one experiences a given moment. States can range from energized and focused to lethargic and anxious. While some states support well-being and productivity, others perpetuate stagnation or distress. Breaking unhelpful states is the first step toward replacing them with ones that align with desired outcomes.

The process of state breaking begins with awareness. One must first recognize when they are caught in a limiting state. This requires attunement to internal signals—racing thoughts, tight muscles, shallow breathing—as well as external cues, such as repetitive behaviors or interactions. For example, noticing a tendency to procrastinate when faced with a challenging task reveals a state of avoidance or fear. Similarly, identifying a pattern of snapping at loved ones under stress highlights a reactive emotional state.

Once a limiting state is identified, the next step is to interrupt it. The human mind and body are highly adaptable, and even small disruptions can shift the momentum of a pattern. Techniques for state breaking vary widely, from physical movements to mental exercises, but all share a common goal: to jolt the system out of its automatic mode and into the present moment.

One of the simplest and most effective methods is physical movement. Changing posture, stretching, or engaging in a burst of activity—such as jumping or shaking out the limbs—disrupts the physical signals that reinforce the current state. For example, standing up and walking briskly can break the lethargy of an unproductive afternoon, while taking a deep, intentional breath can calm the racing heart of anxiety.

Humor is another powerful state breaker. Laughter, even when forced initially, triggers a cascade of physiological and psychological changes that lift mood and perspective. Watching a funny video, recalling a humorous memory, or even practicing a smile can shift a negative state almost instantaneously.

Shifting focus is equally effective. The mind tends to fixate within the bounds of a limiting state, looping through the same thoughts or emotions. Redirecting attention—whether to a new activity, a different sensory input, or a positive memory—breaks this loop. For instance, stepping outside to observe nature or focusing on the texture of an object in your hand can ground you in the present, dissolving the grip of unhelpful thoughts.

Language, both internal and external, plays a critical role in state breaking. Changing the way you speak to yourself—replacing defeatist thoughts like *"I can't do this"* with empowering ones like *"I am figuring this out"*—shifts the mental narrative that sustains the current state. Similarly, speaking aloud affirmations or verbalizing gratitude can create a new emotional tone, breaking the hold of negativity.

Music and sound are potent tools for altering states. Listening to an upbeat song can energize, while calming instrumental music can soothe. Even the act of humming or vocalizing sounds, such as chanting or deep tones, resonates within the body, creating vibrations that disrupt tension and promote relaxation.

Anchoring, discussed earlier, is another valuable technique for state breaking. By activating a positive anchor—a gesture, word, or memory previously associated with an empowering state—you can instantly shift from a limiting state to one of confidence, calm, or joy.

In addition to these immediate techniques, breaking deeper, more entrenched states may require a broader approach. Reflecting on the triggers that lead to certain states provides insight into their origins and patterns. For example, a recurring state of frustration at work might stem from unmet expectations or a lack of boundaries. Addressing these root causes not only breaks the current state but also reduces the likelihood of its recurrence.

State breaking is not just about escaping negative experiences; it is also a way to create momentum for growth and action. When faced with inertia or indecision, a deliberate state break injects energy and focus, propelling you forward. For instance, adopting a power pose—standing tall with hands on hips—can evoke feelings of strength and readiness, making it easier to tackle daunting tasks.

In relationships, state breaking fosters healthier interactions. Conflict often arises when both parties are trapped in reactive states, escalating tension. Introducing a state break—such as pausing the conversation, using humor, or suggesting a change of scenery—can diffuse emotions and create space for constructive dialogue.

While state breaking is a powerful tool, it requires practice to master. The mind and body may resist disruption, clinging to familiar patterns even when they are unhelpful. Persistence and experimentation are key, as different techniques work better for different individuals and situations. Over time, state breaking becomes a natural response to challenges, a habit that supports resilience and adaptability.

It is important to note that state breaking is not about suppressing emotions or denying experiences. Rather, it is a way to create choice—an opportunity to respond intentionally rather than react automatically. By breaking the hold of limiting states, you reclaim agency over how you think, feel, and act.

As you integrate state breaking into your life, its benefits extend beyond immediate relief. The practice fosters a deeper awareness of your emotional and mental landscape, strengthening the connection between intention and action. It empowers you to navigate life's complexities with greater flexibility, transforming challenges into opportunities for growth.

Through state breaking, you unlock the freedom to choose your path moment by moment. You gain the ability to step out of old patterns and into new possibilities, aligning your actions with your goals and values. This practice is not merely a tool for change—it is a celebration of the human capacity for transformation, a reminder that every moment holds the potential for renewal and growth.

Chapter 15
Self-Responsibility

At the heart of personal transformation lies a profound truth: lasting change begins with taking full responsibility for one's life. Self-responsibility is the practice of owning one's thoughts, emotions, actions, and outcomes without shifting blame to external circumstances or other people. It is an act of empowerment, a declaration that the course of life is shaped from within.

To embrace self-responsibility is to recognize the limits of control and the boundless power of choice. While we cannot dictate every event or external force, we retain the ability to choose how we interpret and respond to them. This shift from external dependence to internal accountability transforms victimhood into agency and passivity into purpose.

The journey toward self-responsibility begins with awareness. It requires examining the narratives we tell ourselves about why things are the way they are. Blaming circumstances—*"I would succeed if only I had more time"*—or others—*"They make me so angry"*—shifts accountability outward, relinquishing power. By contrast, self-responsibility reframes these narratives: *"How can I make time for what matters?"* or *"Why am I allowing their actions to control my emotions?"*

This shift in perspective fosters a sense of ownership over life's outcomes. It does not deny external influences or the complexity of challenges but emphasizes the power to choose how to navigate them. For example, financial difficulties might stem from economic conditions, but self-responsibility focuses on actions within one's control—budgeting, seeking new opportunities, or learning new skills—to address them.

Taking responsibility also involves acknowledging the role of beliefs and habits in shaping reality. Limiting beliefs, formed through past experiences or societal conditioning, often operate unnoticed, constraining potential. For instance, believing *"I'm not good at this"* becomes a self-fulfilling prophecy, discouraging effort and reinforcing failure. Self-responsibility challenges these beliefs: *"What evidence supports this? How can I learn and improve?"* This inquiry transforms limitation into possibility.

Similarly, habitual behaviors—whether productive or destructive—arise from choices, often repeated unconsciously. Recognizing this dynamic empowers us to examine habits critically. Are they aligned with our values and goals? If not, what choices can replace them? Self-responsibility turns this reflection into action, fostering intentionality in daily life.

A significant aspect of self-responsibility is emotional accountability. While external events and interactions may trigger emotions, the response to those emotions is a personal choice. Reacting impulsively—yelling in anger, retreating in fear—reinforces patterns that hinder growth. By contrast, responding intentionally—pausing to breathe, expressing feelings constructively—builds emotional resilience and strengthens relationships.

Owning one's emotions does not mean suppressing them. On the contrary, it involves acknowledging and exploring them with curiosity. What is the emotion signaling? What unmet need or unresolved issue lies beneath it? Self-responsibility transforms emotions from barriers into guides, offering insights that support growth.

Critically, self-responsibility does not equate to self-blame. It is not about shouldering undue guilt for every misstep or failure. Blame looks backward, focusing on fault; responsibility looks forward, focusing on solutions. For example, instead of lamenting a missed opportunity, self-responsibility asks, *"What can I do differently next time?"* This forward-thinking mindset fosters learning and progress rather than stagnation.

The practice of self-responsibility also involves setting and maintaining boundaries. Without boundaries, it becomes easy to take on responsibilities that are not ours, leading to burnout or resentment. For instance, trying to fix someone else's problems or overcommitting to tasks outside our capacity erodes personal well-being. Clear boundaries honor both personal needs and mutual respect, creating space for balanced growth.

Another dimension of self-responsibility is accountability to others. While personal growth is an inward journey, its effects ripple outward, influencing relationships and communities. Owning one's actions—apologizing for mistakes, following through on commitments—builds trust and fosters collaboration. This accountability strengthens connections, reinforcing the interdependence of self and others.

Practical tools support the development of self-responsibility. Journaling, for example, provides a structured way to reflect on daily choices, emotions, and outcomes. By documenting thoughts and actions, patterns emerge, revealing areas for growth. Affirmations, such as *"I take ownership of my life"* or *"I have the power to choose my path,"* reinforce the mindset of responsibility, embedding it into daily consciousness.

Visualization is another powerful tool. By imagining oneself navigating challenges with confidence and agency, the mind rehearses new patterns of response. This mental practice builds neural pathways that support real-world application, strengthening the connection between intention and action.

The practice of gratitude also enhances self-responsibility. Acknowledging the positive aspects of life, even amidst difficulty, shifts focus from lack to abundance. This perspective fosters a sense of agency, highlighting the resources and opportunities available for growth.

As self-responsibility becomes a habit, its impact extends beyond personal transformation. It inspires others, modeling a way of being that prioritizes accountability, integrity, and empowerment. This ripple effect creates a culture of responsibility, where individuals and communities thrive together.

Embracing self-responsibility is not without its challenges. It requires confronting uncomfortable truths, letting go of excuses, and making choices that demand effort and courage. Yet, it is through this process that true freedom is found—the freedom to shape one's destiny, regardless of external circumstances.

Ultimately, self-responsibility is an act of self-respect. It acknowledges the inherent power within to create, to grow, and to overcome. By taking ownership of life's journey, we honor our potential, transforming challenges into stepping stones and intentions into realities.

Through self-responsibility, the narrative of life shifts from *"Why is this happening to me?"* to *"What can I do about it?"* This shift is not merely a change in words but a profound transformation in perspective, one that empowers us to live with purpose, resilience, and authenticity.

Chapter 16
Values and Purpose

At the core of every transformative journey lies a compass: the deeply held values that guide decisions, shape actions, and define meaning. These values are not merely abstract ideals but the foundation of a purposeful life, the principles that align who we are with what we do. When we live in accordance with our values, we experience authenticity, fulfillment, and clarity. Conversely, when we stray from them, life often feels fragmented or directionless. To identify and embrace these values is to unlock the transformative power of purpose.

Values are the intrinsic beliefs that determine what matters most to us. They act as internal signposts, pointing toward the life we wish to create. For some, values might include integrity, creativity, or family; for others, they may center on growth, freedom, or connection. Each person's values are unique, reflecting their experiences, aspirations, and individuality.

The journey of uncovering these values begins with introspection. Often, values operate beneath conscious awareness, influencing decisions without being explicitly recognized. Reflecting on pivotal moments in life—times of joy, pride, or challenge—provides clues to what we truly hold dear. Ask yourself: *What moments felt deeply meaningful to me? What principles guided my actions in those times?* Patterns begin to emerge, revealing the values at the heart of your identity.

Another approach is to examine moments of discontent or frustration. These experiences often highlight where values are being compromised. For instance, persistent dissatisfaction in a job might point to a value of creativity stifled by routine, or tension in a relationship might signal a value of respect being unmet. These reflections illuminate areas where alignment with values is lacking, offering opportunities for realignment.

Once values are identified, the next step is to prioritize them. While many things may feel important, living in alignment requires clarity about what matters most. Consider ranking your values or grouping them into categories, distinguishing between core values—those that define your essence—and secondary values that support them. This hierarchy creates a clearer framework for decision-making and goal-setting.

Purpose emerges from this alignment of values. It is the expression of what gives life meaning, the bridge between inner beliefs and outward action. While values define what matters, purpose answers the question: *How can I live these values in a way that contributes to the world?* For example, a value of compassion might lead to a purpose of helping others, or a value of innovation might inspire a purpose of creating solutions to complex problems.

Clarifying purpose involves envisioning the impact you wish to have. What legacy do you want to leave? What problems do you feel called to solve? What brings you a sense of contribution and fulfillment? Purpose need not be grand or universal; it can be as simple as nurturing meaningful relationships or as ambitious as driving societal change. The key is that it resonates deeply with your values and aspirations.

Living in alignment with values and purpose requires consistency and intentionality. It involves making choices that honor these principles, even when they are difficult or inconvenient. For instance, upholding a value of honesty might mean having a challenging conversation, while prioritizing a purpose of personal growth might require stepping outside your comfort zone. These choices reinforce integrity, building a life that reflects who you truly are.

Challenges inevitably arise in this process. External pressures—expectations from society, family, or peers—often pull us away from our values, creating tension and doubt.

Navigating these pressures requires courage and self-awareness, a willingness to prioritize inner truth over external approval. Journaling, meditation, or seeking guidance from mentors can help maintain clarity and resolve during these moments.

Boundaries also play a vital role in preserving alignment. Without clear boundaries, it becomes easy to compromise values in the face of demands or distractions. Setting limits on time, energy, or commitments ensures that actions remain focused on what truly matters. For example, saying no to a project that conflicts with a value of family time reinforces both the value and the sense of purpose it supports.

Purpose is not static; it evolves as life unfolds. Major life transitions—a new career, a shift in relationships, or personal growth—often prompt a reevaluation of values and purpose. Embracing this evolution is not a betrayal of past beliefs but a natural progression, reflecting the dynamic nature of human experience. Regularly revisiting your values ensures they remain aligned with who you are becoming.

The benefits of living in alignment are profound. Decisions become clearer, guided by the framework of values and purpose. Relationships deepen, grounded in authenticity and mutual respect. Challenges, rather than derailing, become opportunities to reaffirm commitment to what matters. Most importantly, life gains a sense of coherence and meaning, as actions reflect the deepest truths of the self.

In addition to personal transformation, living with purpose inspires others. A life lived in alignment radiates integrity and conviction, encouraging those around you to reflect on their own values. This ripple effect extends beyond the individual, fostering a culture of authenticity and intentionality.

Practical tools support this alignment. Visualization, for example, helps connect values to daily life. Imagine a day lived fully in alignment: What choices would you make? How would you interact with others? What emotions would dominate? This exercise bridges the gap between abstract principles and concrete actions, making alignment tangible.

Affirmations also reinforce alignment, anchoring values and purpose in daily consciousness. Statements like *"I live with integrity and intention"* or *"My actions reflect my deepest values"* serve as reminders of what matters most. Repeating these affirmations regularly strengthens their influence, embedding them into thought and behavior.

Finally, gratitude amplifies the experience of alignment. Acknowledging moments where values are honored or purpose is fulfilled cultivates a sense of fulfillment and motivation. For example, reflecting on a conversation where you upheld a value of respect or celebrating a project aligned with your purpose reinforces the joy of living authentically.

Values and purpose are not destinations but guiding stars, illuminating the path toward a life of meaning and fulfillment. By aligning actions with these principles, you create a life that is not only intentional but also deeply satisfying. Through this practice, you embrace the transformative power of authenticity, living not according to what is expected but according to what is true.

In this alignment, transformation becomes inevitable. The life you create mirrors the essence of who you are, reflecting a harmony between inner beliefs and outward expression. It is in this harmony that the greatest potential for growth, connection, and contribution is found, a testament to the power of values and purpose to shape a life of extraordinary depth and meaning.

Chapter 17
Focus and Direction

In the journey of transformation, clarity of focus and direction serves as a guiding light, cutting through the noise of distractions and doubts. Focus concentrates energy, while direction provides a sense of purpose and trajectory. Together, they create the foundation for meaningful action and sustained progress, aligning intentions with outcomes.

Focus begins with the ability to direct attention intentionally. In an age of constant information and competing demands, the mind is often scattered, pulled in multiple directions at once. This fragmentation diminishes productivity, clarity, and fulfillment. Reclaiming focus requires cultivating awareness of where attention is spent and redirecting it toward what truly matters.

A key step in developing focus is identifying priorities. Not all tasks or goals carry equal weight, and clarity about what deserves attention is essential. Ask yourself: *What are the most important outcomes I want to achieve? What actions align with my values and purpose?* By distinguishing between urgent but trivial tasks and those that contribute to long-term growth, focus becomes a tool for intentional living rather than mere reaction.

To sharpen focus, mindfulness serves as a powerful ally. Mindfulness is the practice of anchoring awareness in the present moment, free from judgment or distraction. By observing thoughts and sensations without attachment, mindfulness cultivates mental discipline and clarity. For instance, taking a few minutes each day to focus on the breath or engage in mindful observation of surroundings strengthens the ability to stay present and intentional in daily life.

Equally important is managing external distractions. Digital devices, notifications, and multitasking often fragment attention, creating a cycle of constant interruption. Establishing boundaries—such as setting specific times for checking email or silencing unnecessary alerts—protects focus. Creating a dedicated, clutter-free workspace further minimizes distractions, fostering an environment that supports sustained attention.

While focus sharpens the present moment, direction charts the path ahead. Direction is the clarity of where you want to go and why it matters. Without direction, effort can become aimless, leading to frustration and stagnation. Setting clear goals bridges the gap between intention and achievement, providing a roadmap for progress.

Effective goal-setting involves specificity, measurability, and alignment with values. A vague aspiration like *"I want to be healthier"* lacks actionable steps and focus. By contrast, a specific goal such as *"I will exercise for 30 minutes, five days a week"* creates clarity and accountability. This precision not only clarifies the goal but also makes progress easier to track and celebrate.

The SMART framework—Specific, Measurable, Achievable, Relevant, and Time-bound—provides a structure for setting effective goals. For example, a goal of *"I will complete a professional certification within six months"* meets all SMART criteria, offering a clear and actionable objective.

Visualizing the desired outcome enhances both focus and direction. By vividly imagining the end result—whether it is a successful project, a personal milestone, or a state of well-being—you create a mental blueprint that guides effort. Visualization not only clarifies the goal but also strengthens motivation, as the mind begins to associate the vision with reality.

Breaking large goals into smaller, manageable steps further supports focus and direction. Each step serves as a milestone, building momentum and confidence. For example, a goal of writing a book can be divided into chapters, with each chapter further broken down into daily writing sessions. This approach transforms daunting ambitions into achievable tasks, maintaining focus while ensuring steady progress.

Consistency is crucial in maintaining focus and direction. While motivation often fluctuates, discipline sustains effort over time. Establishing routines and habits that align with your goals reinforces consistency. For instance, dedicating a specific time each day to work on a priority project creates a rhythm that minimizes the need for constant decision-making about when to act.

Flexibility complements consistency, allowing for adjustments when circumstances change. Life is dynamic, and rigid adherence to a plan can lead to frustration when unexpected challenges arise. Revisiting and refining goals ensures that they remain relevant and achievable, preserving direction without sacrificing adaptability.

Obstacles are inevitable on any path, but focus and direction provide the resilience to navigate them. Instead of becoming discouraged by setbacks, view them as opportunities for reflection and growth. Ask: *What can I learn from this? How can I adjust my approach to move forward?* This mindset transforms challenges into stepping stones, reinforcing commitment to the journey.

Reflection also plays a vital role in sustaining focus and direction. Regularly evaluating progress—whether through journaling, discussions with mentors, or quiet introspection—ensures alignment with your goals and values. Celebrate achievements, no matter how small, as markers of progress. Simultaneously, identify areas for improvement, using them as opportunities to refine your path.

Balancing focus and direction requires attention to both short-term actions and long-term vision. While it is important to remain present and engaged in daily tasks, maintaining sight of the larger purpose prevents getting lost in minutiae. Periodically stepping back to review the broader trajectory ensures that actions remain aligned with meaningful outcomes.

In relationships, focus and direction foster deeper connections. Being fully present during conversations—listening without distraction, responding with intention—strengthens bonds. Shared goals within partnerships or teams create a sense of purpose and collaboration, aligning efforts toward mutual success.

As focus and direction become integral to your life, they cultivate a sense of mastery and fulfillment. The ability to concentrate on what matters, coupled with a clear vision of where you are headed, transforms effort into achievement. This alignment brings a profound sense of purpose, as actions reflect values and aspirations.

Ultimately, focus and direction are not static qualities but dynamic practices, honed through intention and effort. They evolve with you, adapting to new challenges, opportunities, and insights. By cultivating these skills, you create a life that is not only productive but also deeply meaningful—a life where every step is taken with clarity, intention, and purpose.

Through the synergy of focus and direction, transformation becomes more than a possibility; it becomes a lived reality. The path ahead is illuminated by intention, and each step forward reinforces the truth that a purposeful life is within reach, waiting to be shaped by your choices and vision.

Chapter 18
Emotional Detachment

Emotions are the pulse of the human experience, coloring every thought, decision, and interaction. They enrich life with depth and meaning but can also entangle us in patterns of pain, fear, or attachment. Emotional detachment is not the absence of feeling; it is the art of releasing emotional reactions that tether us to the past or cloud our perspective. This practice fosters clarity, resilience, and freedom, enabling us to engage with life authentically and purposefully.

Detachment begins with understanding the nature of emotional attachment. At its core, attachment arises when we become overly invested in a specific outcome, relationship, or identity. This investment often stems from fear—the fear of loss, failure, or change. For example, clinging to a past relationship out of fear of loneliness, or obsessing over a missed opportunity, creates emotional weight that hinders growth.

The first step toward detachment is awareness. Recognizing when and where attachments occur provides the foundation for change. This requires mindful observation of your emotional responses. When you feel a strong reaction—whether anger, sadness, or anxiety—pause and ask: *What am I holding onto? What story or expectation is fueling this emotion?* This reflection reveals the attachments shaping your inner world.

Releasing these attachments does not mean dismissing or suppressing emotions. On the contrary, it involves fully experiencing and acknowledging them without letting them control your actions or self-concept. This distinction is key: emotions are not enemies to be defeated but messages to be understood. For instance, feelings of jealousy might reveal unmet needs for recognition or connection. By addressing the root cause rather than clinging to the emotion itself, detachment becomes a tool for insight and growth.

Mindfulness is a powerful practice for cultivating detachment. By anchoring attention in the present moment, mindfulness creates space between the self and the emotion. Imagine sitting by a river, watching emotions flow past like leaves on the water. Instead of being swept away by the current, you observe with curiosity and compassion. This perspective fosters a sense of calm and presence, even in the midst of turmoil.

Another effective technique is reframing. Attachments often stem from rigid expectations or beliefs about how life *should* be. Reframing involves shifting these perspectives to embrace flexibility and acceptance. For example, instead of lamenting a setback as a failure, view it as an opportunity for growth. This shift not only reduces emotional intensity but also aligns your mindset with resilience and possibility.

Detachment also requires letting go of control. Many attachments are rooted in the desire to control outcomes or avoid uncertainty. Yet, life is inherently unpredictable, and clinging to control often leads to frustration and stress. Surrendering to the flow of life—trusting that you can navigate challenges without needing to dominate them—fosters a sense of freedom and adaptability. This surrender is not passive resignation but active engagement with what is, rather than what might or should be.

Boundaries play a crucial role in emotional detachment, particularly in relationships. While connections with others are vital, over-identification with their emotions or actions can blur the lines between empathy and enmeshment. Setting boundaries ensures that you remain supportive without absorbing others' feelings as your own. For example, offering understanding to a friend in distress does not mean taking responsibility for their choices or emotions. This balance preserves your emotional well-being while fostering healthy relationships.

Physical practices, such as deep breathing or progressive muscle relaxation, support detachment by calming the body's stress response. Emotions often manifest physically—tightness in the chest, clenched fists, or a racing heart. By addressing these physical cues, you create a pathway to emotional release. For instance, taking slow, intentional breaths during moments of anger or anxiety signals the nervous system to relax, breaking the cycle of reactive attachment.

Visualization can also aid in detachment. Imagine the emotion or attachment as a cord connecting you to a specific person, situation, or belief. Visualize yourself gently cutting the cord, releasing the energy that binds you. This symbolic act reinforces the intention to let go, creating a sense of closure and freedom.

Gratitude serves as a powerful counterbalance to attachment. By focusing on what you have rather than what you fear losing, gratitude shifts attention from lack to abundance. For example, appreciating the lessons of a past experience rather than mourning its end transforms attachment into acceptance. This practice cultivates a mindset of openness and trust in life's unfolding.

Detachment also involves self-compassion. Letting go of attachments, particularly deeply ingrained ones, can be challenging and uncomfortable. Offering yourself kindness during this process—acknowledging the difficulty without self-criticism—fosters resilience and perseverance. Remember that detachment is not a one-time act but an ongoing practice, one that deepens with intention and patience.

While detachment centers on releasing unhelpful attachments, it does not mean disengagement from life. On the contrary, detachment enhances engagement by removing the filters of fear and expectation. It allows you to approach situations with clarity and presence, unburdened by past narratives or future anxieties. For instance, detachment from the need for approval frees you to express yourself authentically, deepening your connections and creativity.

As you integrate detachment into your life, its benefits extend beyond emotional well-being. Detachment fosters greater clarity in decision-making, as choices are guided by values rather than reactive emotions. It strengthens resilience, enabling you to navigate challenges with grace and adaptability. Most importantly, it nurtures a sense of inner freedom, the ability to live fully and authentically regardless of external circumstances.

Ultimately, emotional detachment is an act of liberation. It frees you from the chains of past wounds, unfulfilled expectations, and fear-based attachments, creating space for growth, joy, and peace. Through this practice, you discover that the essence of who you are is not defined by what you hold onto but by your capacity to let go and embrace the present moment.

In mastering emotional detachment, you reclaim the power to shape your inner world. The result is not indifference but profound connection—a connection to yourself, to others, and to the flow of life, unclouded by attachment and enriched by the clarity of freedom.

Chapter 19
Mirroring Technique

Human connection thrives on understanding, and understanding is deepened by rapport. The mirroring technique, a cornerstone of Neuro-Linguistic Programming (NLP), is a method that fosters connection and trust by subtly reflecting the behaviors, emotions, and communication styles of others. This technique, when practiced with authenticity and intention, enhances personal and professional relationships, creating harmony and mutual respect.

At its essence, mirroring is the practice of aligning with another person's verbal and nonverbal cues to create a sense of familiarity and comfort. It is rooted in the natural human tendency to connect with those who seem similar to us. When two individuals share synchronized behaviors—whether in posture, tone, or rhythm—a subconscious bond forms, making communication more effective and relationships more meaningful.

The power of mirroring lies in its subtlety. It is not about imitation or mimicry but about resonance. Done skillfully, mirroring creates a flow of interaction where both parties feel seen, heard, and understood. For example, matching the energy of someone's enthusiasm in a conversation conveys engagement, while adopting a calm demeanor when speaking to someone anxious signals reassurance.

To begin using the mirroring technique, awareness is key. Observe the other person's body language: their posture, gestures, and facial expressions. Note their tone of voice, pace of speech, and choice of words. Pay attention not just to what they are saying but how they are expressing it. For instance, are their movements expansive or reserved? Is their speech rapid or deliberate? These cues provide insight into their emotional state and communication style.

Once these patterns are recognized, gently align with them. If someone is leaning forward in an animated conversation, you might lean in slightly to show interest. If their speech is slow and deliberate, match their pacing in your response. This alignment creates a rhythm of interaction that fosters rapport, as the other person subconsciously perceives you as being "in sync" with them.

Mirroring extends beyond body language and speech to emotional resonance. Empathy plays a central role in this aspect of the technique. By tuning into the other person's feelings, you reflect not just their outward expressions but the emotions underlying them. For example, if someone shares a personal struggle, mirroring their tone and offering empathetic responses like *"That sounds really challenging"* demonstrates understanding and care.

The practice also involves adapting communication styles to match the other person's preferences. Some individuals are highly visual, describing their thoughts with phrases like *"I see what you mean"* or *"It looks clear to me."* Others may be more auditory, using expressions like *"That sounds right"* or *"I hear you."* Adopting similar language creates a deeper connection by speaking in terms that resonate with their cognitive patterns.

Timing is critical in mirroring. Effective mirroring occurs in real time, subtly and naturally. Overly delayed or exaggerated attempts can feel forced, breaking the flow of interaction. For instance, if someone crosses their arms, mirroring them minutes later would seem disjointed. Instead, align smoothly and adjust as the conversation evolves.

While the technique is powerful, it must be grounded in authenticity. Mirroring is not about manipulation or insincerity but about fostering genuine connection. The intention should always be to build understanding and rapport, not to control or deceive. Authentic mirroring comes from a place of respect and empathy, reinforcing the foundation of trust.

The mirroring technique is particularly effective in diffusing tension and resolving conflict. When disagreements arise, reflecting the other person's tone and posture can signal openness and willingness to understand. For example, if someone raises their voice in frustration, maintaining a calm but attentive demeanor helps de-escalate the situation. Similarly, restating their concerns in their own words—*"I hear that you're frustrated because..."*—validates their feelings and paves the way for constructive dialogue.

In professional settings, mirroring enhances collaboration and influence. Building rapport with colleagues, clients, or team members creates a foundation of mutual respect that facilitates problem-solving and decision-making. For instance, during negotiations, aligning with the other party's communication style fosters trust, increasing the likelihood of finding common ground.

In personal relationships, mirroring deepens emotional intimacy. By reflecting a partner's expressions and emotions, you create a safe space for vulnerability and connection. For example, mirroring excitement about a shared milestone or empathizing with their challenges through matching tone and gestures strengthens the bond between you.

Practicing the mirroring technique requires patience and self-awareness. It begins with small, deliberate efforts—matching a gesture or tone here, aligning with a pace of speech there—and gradually becomes second nature. The more you practice, the more intuitive the process becomes, allowing for seamless and authentic interactions.

It is important to be mindful of individual differences when using the technique. Not everyone responds to mirroring in the same way, and cultural or personal preferences may influence its effectiveness. Sensitivity to these factors ensures that mirroring is used respectfully and appropriately, enhancing rather than hindering connection.

Mirroring also fosters personal growth. By observing and reflecting others, you become more attuned to your own communication patterns, gaining insight into how you are perceived. This self-awareness strengthens your ability to adapt and connect across diverse contexts, making you a more effective communicator and empathetic listener.

Ultimately, the mirroring technique is not just about connection—it is about harmony. It bridges gaps in understanding, transforms interactions, and nurtures relationships, creating a flow of communication that feels natural and meaningful. Through this practice, you cultivate not only stronger bonds with others but also a deeper understanding of yourself.

In mastering the art of mirroring, you unlock a powerful tool for building trust, fostering collaboration, and enriching relationships. It is a testament to the transformative power of empathy and connection, a reminder that understanding begins not with speaking but with listening and reflecting.

Chapter 20
Emotional Intelligence

Emotional intelligence (EI) is the bridge between self-awareness and meaningful interaction with others, a skill that shapes both personal transformation and relational success. It encompasses the ability to understand, manage, and express emotions effectively while navigating the emotions of those around us with empathy and skill. Mastering emotional intelligence transforms how we engage with challenges, relationships, and growth, creating a foundation for lasting change.

At its core, emotional intelligence is built on five interconnected pillars: self-awareness, self-regulation, motivation, empathy, and social skills. Together, these elements form a dynamic framework that empowers individuals to align their internal world with their external actions.

Self-awareness is the cornerstone of emotional intelligence. It involves recognizing and understanding one's emotions as they arise, along with the thoughts and behaviors they influence. Cultivating self-awareness requires observing emotional patterns without judgment, asking questions like: *What am I feeling? Why am I feeling this way? How does this emotion affect my choices?* Journaling, mindfulness, and meditation are valuable tools for developing this skill, as they create space for reflection and clarity.

Self-regulation builds on self-awareness by fostering the ability to manage emotions constructively. It does not mean suppressing emotions but rather channeling them in ways that support growth and well-being. For instance, rather than reacting impulsively to anger, self-regulation involves pausing, identifying its source, and choosing a measured response. Techniques such as deep breathing, visualization, or reframing help create this pause, transforming emotional reactivity into intentional action.

Motivation, the third pillar, ties emotional intelligence to purpose and resilience. Intrinsic motivation—driven by personal values and aspirations—sustains effort even in the face of setbacks. Reflecting on what inspires you, setting meaningful goals, and celebrating progress foster a sense of purpose that aligns emotions with action. For example, when pursuing a challenging project, reconnecting with the value it represents can reignite determination and focus.

Empathy extends emotional intelligence outward, enabling us to understand and resonate with the emotions of others. It requires active listening, attunement to nonverbal cues, and a genuine desire to connect. Empathy bridges differences, creating a sense of shared humanity that deepens relationships and fosters trust. By asking open-ended questions like *"How are you feeling?"* or offering validation—*"I understand why this is important to you"*—we demonstrate care and openness, enhancing emotional connection.

Social skills, the final pillar, translate emotional intelligence into effective interaction. They include clear communication, conflict resolution, collaboration, and the ability to inspire or influence others positively. Social skills depend on the interplay of all other pillars, integrating self-awareness, regulation, motivation, and empathy into relational contexts. For example, resolving a workplace disagreement might involve regulating personal frustration, empathizing with the other party's perspective, and finding solutions that align with shared goals.

While each pillar is distinct, they function as a cohesive whole. Strengthening one enhances the others, creating a cycle of growth that expands both personal and interpersonal capacity. For instance, improved self-regulation fosters greater empathy by reducing emotional interference, while heightened motivation enhances social skills through clear, purpose-driven communication.

The benefits of emotional intelligence are far-reaching. On a personal level, it supports mental health by reducing stress, improving resilience, and fostering self-acceptance. Professionally, it enhances leadership, teamwork, and adaptability, qualities that drive success in dynamic environments. In relationships, emotional intelligence deepens connection, creating bonds rooted in understanding and mutual respect.

Developing emotional intelligence requires intention and practice. Begin with self-awareness by dedicating time to reflect on your emotional landscape. Pay attention to triggers—situations or interactions that evoke strong emotions—and explore their underlying causes. For example, recurring feelings of insecurity might stem from a belief about inadequacy, while frequent frustration may point to unmet needs or values. Identifying these patterns provides a foundation for growth.

Self-regulation practices follow naturally from this awareness. Experiment with techniques that suit your needs, such as grounding exercises to manage anxiety or reframing thoughts to shift perspective. For example, if a colleague's criticism triggers defensiveness, reframing the feedback as an opportunity to learn fosters a constructive response.

Motivation thrives on clarity of purpose. Regularly revisit your goals and the values they reflect, using them as a compass for decision-making. Visualizing success or creating a vision board can reinforce this alignment, keeping intrinsic motivation at the forefront.

Empathy grows through active engagement with others. Practice listening without interrupting or formulating responses in advance. Observe nonverbal signals—posture, tone, facial expressions—that reveal emotions beyond words. Cultivate curiosity about others' experiences, asking questions that invite deeper sharing, and approach differences with openness rather than judgment.

Social skills are honed through deliberate interaction. Seek opportunities to collaborate, mediate, or lead in ways that align with your emotional intelligence. For instance, during team discussions, balancing assertiveness with empathy fosters both clarity and cohesion. Similarly, offering constructive feedback with sensitivity strengthens trust and communication.

Challenges in developing emotional intelligence are inevitable. Emotional habits, deeply ingrained over time, resist change. Moments of failure—reacting impulsively, misunderstanding others, or struggling to stay motivated—are natural and provide opportunities for growth. Approach these moments with self-compassion, viewing them as part of the learning process rather than setbacks.

Feedback from trusted peers, mentors, or coaches accelerates growth. Others often see patterns we overlook, offering valuable insights into how we engage emotionally. Their perspective, combined with self-reflection, creates a more comprehensive understanding of strengths and areas for improvement.

Ultimately, emotional intelligence is not a fixed trait but an evolving practice. It grows with effort and intention, adapting to new experiences and challenges. Over time, it becomes a way of being, a natural integration of emotional awareness, regulation, and connection that enhances every aspect of life.

In mastering emotional intelligence, you discover the power to navigate your inner world and the complexity of relationships with grace and authenticity. It is a skill that empowers you to align emotions with purpose, foster understanding, and create connections that inspire growth and transformation. Through this practice, you cultivate not only a deeper connection to yourself but also to the world around you, embodying the essence of emotional and relational mastery.

Chapter 21
Overcoming Fear

Fear is a primal and pervasive emotion, designed to protect and preserve us from danger. Yet, in the context of modern life, fear often transcends its original purpose, creating barriers that hinder growth, stifle creativity, and limit potential. Overcoming fear is not about erasing it; it is about transforming it into a tool for self-discovery and progress. By addressing fear with curiosity and courage, it becomes a stepping stone rather than an obstacle on the path of transformation.

The first step in overcoming fear is understanding its nature. Fear often arises from uncertainty, vulnerability, or the anticipation of loss. While some fears are tangible—rooted in real threats—many are abstract, products of the mind's imagination. These intangible fears, such as fear of failure, rejection, or inadequacy, often carry disproportionate weight, influencing decisions and actions even when the perceived danger is minimal.

Awareness is the foundation of transformation. Recognizing fear as it arises, rather than suppressing or ignoring it, creates the opportunity for change. This requires mindfulness—pausing to observe the physical sensations, thoughts, and emotions associated with fear. Ask yourself: *What am I afraid of? What is the worst that could happen? What am I truly protecting myself from?* These questions illuminate the roots of fear, turning it from an amorphous force into a specific challenge.

Once fear is identified, reframing it becomes possible. Fear, at its core, signals the boundaries of comfort. Rather than viewing it as a barrier, consider it a guidepost, indicating areas where growth is possible. For example, the fear of public speaking might reflect the potential for increased confidence and communication skills. Reframing fear in this way shifts its role from adversary to ally, aligning it with your goals rather than opposing them.

Another powerful technique for overcoming fear is gradual exposure. Facing fears incrementally, in controlled and manageable steps, desensitizes the mind to their impact. For instance, someone afraid of social interactions might start by engaging in brief conversations with strangers, gradually increasing the complexity and duration of interactions over time. Each small success builds confidence, reducing fear's hold and expanding the boundaries of comfort.

Visualization plays a crucial role in this process. By vividly imagining yourself confronting and overcoming a fear, you create a mental rehearsal that strengthens neural pathways associated with success. For instance, if you fear failure in a project, visualize yourself navigating challenges with resilience and ultimately achieving your goal. This practice not only reduces anxiety but also primes the mind for action, creating a sense of familiarity with the desired outcome.

Breathing techniques provide an immediate and effective way to manage fear's physiological effects. Fear often triggers a fight-or-flight response, marked by rapid breathing, increased heart rate, and tension. Deep, intentional breathing counteracts this response, calming the nervous system and restoring clarity. Practices such as diaphragmatic breathing or the 4-7-8 technique (inhaling for four counts, holding for seven, exhaling for eight) create a sense of control and grounding.

Language also shapes how we engage with fear. Words like *"I can't"* or *"I'm terrified"* reinforce fear's power, embedding it in identity. Replacing these phrases with empowering alternatives—*"I'm learning to face this"* or *"This is challenging, but I'm capable"*—reframes the narrative, reducing fear's grip. Affirmations, such as *"I am stronger than my fears"* or *"I grow through challenges,"* further reinforce resilience and determination.

Support from others accelerates the process of overcoming fear. Sharing fears with trusted friends, mentors, or support groups normalizes the experience, reducing its stigma and isolation. Their encouragement, perspective, and advice provide a foundation of reassurance, making fear feel less insurmountable. Collaborative exploration of solutions often reveals strategies and insights that might not arise in isolation.

While fear is often perceived as a weakness, it holds valuable lessons. Exploring the deeper beliefs and experiences underlying fear uncovers patterns that shape behavior and thought. For instance, fear of rejection might stem from past experiences of exclusion, while fear of failure may reflect perfectionist tendencies. Addressing these root causes transforms fear from a symptom into a source of self-awareness, fostering healing and growth.

It is important to acknowledge that overcoming fear is not a linear process. Progress often involves setbacks, moments when fear resurfaces despite previous efforts. These moments are not failures but opportunities to deepen resilience and recommit to the journey. Approaching them with self-compassion—recognizing that growth is an iterative process—fosters perseverance and trust in your ability to navigate challenges.

In addition to individual fears, societal and cultural influences often amplify fear. Expectations, judgments, and comparisons create external pressures that reinforce internal anxieties. Developing a strong sense of self, rooted in values and purpose, counters these influences, reducing their impact. By aligning actions with personal truth rather than external validation, you reclaim agency over your choices and emotions.

As fear diminishes, its transformation becomes evident. What once felt paralyzing now serves as a reminder of courage and progress. The lessons learned through overcoming fear extend to other areas of life, creating a ripple effect of confidence and empowerment. Relationships deepen, as vulnerability is embraced rather than avoided. Opportunities expand, as fear no longer dictates the scope of action.

Ultimately, overcoming fear is an act of liberation. It frees you from the confines of doubt and hesitation, revealing the boundless potential within. Through this practice, fear evolves from a force that limits into a force that fuels, guiding you toward growth, discovery, and fulfillment.

In mastering fear, you discover that it is not the absence of fear that defines courage, but the willingness to act despite it. Each step taken in the face of fear strengthens your resolve, transforming it into a partner on the journey of transformation. In this partnership, fear no longer holds you back—it propels you forward, toward a life of authenticity, possibility, and purpose.

Chapter 22
The Power of Gratitude

Gratitude is a quiet yet profound force, one that reshapes how we perceive the world and our place within it. It is more than a fleeting feeling of thankfulness—it is a practice, a mindset, and a transformative lens through which life gains depth and meaning. By cultivating gratitude, we learn to focus on abundance rather than lack, resilience rather than hardship, and connection rather than isolation. It becomes a cornerstone of personal transformation, fostering well-being, growth, and authentic joy.

Gratitude begins with awareness—the conscious act of noticing and appreciating the positive aspects of life. These aspects can range from the grand to the seemingly insignificant: the support of loved ones, the warmth of sunlight, or even the quiet satisfaction of completing a task. Each moment of recognition strengthens the habit of gratitude, rewiring the mind to seek the good in every situation.

This practice counters the brain's natural negativity bias, an evolutionary tendency to focus on threats and challenges. While this bias once ensured survival, it now often skews our perception, amplifying stress and dissatisfaction. Gratitude interrupts this pattern, redirecting attention toward what is working, what is beautiful, and what is meaningful. Over time, this shift cultivates a more balanced and positive outlook.

To begin fostering gratitude, journaling is a powerful tool. Setting aside a few minutes each day to list things you are grateful for creates a structured space for reflection. The practice can be as simple as noting three things you appreciated that day—a kind gesture, a moment of laughter, or a personal accomplishment.

This consistency anchors gratitude in daily life, making it a habit rather than an occasional thought.

Another practice is expressing gratitude to others. Relationships deepen when we take the time to acknowledge the impact of those around us. A heartfelt thank-you, whether in person, through a written note, or even a brief message, strengthens bonds and fosters mutual appreciation. For example, telling a colleague, *"I really appreciate your help on that project—it made a big difference,"* not only uplifts them but also reinforces the connection between you.

Gratitude is not limited to positive experiences; it can also arise from challenges. Difficulties, while uncomfortable, often carry lessons and opportunities for growth. Reflecting on these hidden gifts transforms adversity into a source of strength and wisdom. For instance, a failed endeavor might teach resilience, while a conflict could reveal the value of honest communication. By practicing gratitude for these lessons, you reframe hardship as an integral part of the journey.

Visualization enhances the practice of gratitude. Take a moment to close your eyes and vividly imagine a person, place, or experience you are grateful for. Engage your senses: recall the sights, sounds, and emotions associated with the memory. This immersive exercise amplifies the feeling of gratitude, making it more tangible and impactful. For example, visualizing a cherished family gathering might evoke warmth, connection, and joy, deepening your appreciation for those relationships.

Gratitude also connects us to the present moment. Often, the mind is consumed by thoughts of the past or worries about the future, pulling attention away from the here and now. Gratitude grounds us, redirecting focus to what is immediately before us. This mindfulness fosters a sense of contentment, as we learn to appreciate life as it unfolds rather than waiting for perfection.

The practice of gratitude extends beyond the self, influencing the world around us. When gratitude becomes a way of life, it radiates outward, inspiring others to adopt the same perspective. Acts of kindness, expressions of appreciation, and a positive presence create a ripple effect, contributing to a culture of gratitude in communities, workplaces, and families.

Despite its simplicity, the practice of gratitude is not always easy. During periods of stress, loss, or uncertainty, finding reasons to be grateful can feel challenging, even impossible. In these moments, it is important to start small. Acknowledge even the tiniest blessings: the comfort of a warm drink, the resilience of your own breath, or the opportunity to begin anew each day. These small acknowledgments build a foundation for gratitude, even in the face of difficulty.

Gratitude is also a practice of humility. It reminds us that we are interconnected, that much of what we experience and achieve is made possible by the contributions of others. Recognizing this interdependence fosters a sense of belonging and reduces feelings of isolation. For instance, reflecting on the countless individuals involved in creating a simple meal—from farmers to cooks—reveals the intricate web of connection that sustains us.

The benefits of gratitude are far-reaching. Psychologically, it reduces stress, enhances mood, and fosters resilience. Physically, studies have linked gratitude to improved sleep, lower blood pressure, and stronger immune function. Socially, it strengthens relationships, deepens trust, and promotes empathy. These effects are not fleeting; they compound over time, creating a foundation for long-term well-being.

Incorporating gratitude into daily rituals reinforces its presence in your life. Begin the day with a gratitude-focused meditation, reflecting on what you appreciate before the day's demands take hold. End the day by reviewing moments of gratitude, no matter how small. These rituals create a rhythm that weaves gratitude into the fabric of your life.

As gratitude becomes second nature, its impact transcends the individual. It reshapes how you engage with the world, fostering a mindset of abundance and generosity. Instead of viewing life through the lens of what is missing, you begin to see what is already present—and how much more is possible.

Gratitude becomes not just a reaction to life's gifts but a catalyst for creating and sharing those gifts.

Ultimately, the power of gratitude lies in its simplicity and universality. It requires no special tools or circumstances, only the willingness to pause, notice, and appreciate. Through this practice, you transform your relationship with yourself, others, and the world, discovering that the path to fulfillment begins not with seeking more but with appreciating what is already here.

In mastering gratitude, you uncover a profound truth: that life, in all its imperfection, is a gift. This perspective does not ignore challenges but embraces them, finding beauty and meaning in every experience. Gratitude is not an endpoint but a way of being, a continuous unfolding of appreciation that enriches every moment and empowers transformation.

Chapter 23
Self-Sabotage

Self-sabotage is a quiet adversary, one that operates from within, often unseen and unacknowledged. It is the act of undermining one's own goals, desires, or progress, driven by fears, doubts, or unresolved beliefs. For many, the most formidable obstacles are not external challenges but the internal patterns that hold them back. Understanding and overcoming self-sabotage is essential for personal transformation, as it allows individuals to unlock their full potential and align their actions with their aspirations.

Self-sabotage often manifests in subtle ways: procrastination, perfectionism, indecision, or avoidance. These behaviors, though seemingly minor, accumulate over time, creating significant barriers to growth. At its core, self-sabotage arises from a conflict between conscious goals and subconscious fears. For example, while consciously striving for success, a fear of failure might lead to procrastination, ensuring that success remains out of reach.

The first step in addressing self-sabotage is awareness. Recognizing the behaviors and patterns that derail progress is essential. Begin by reflecting on moments where you felt stuck, frustrated, or unfulfilled. Ask yourself: *What actions or inactions contributed to this outcome? What beliefs or emotions were driving these choices?* Journaling can be particularly effective for identifying recurring themes and gaining clarity.

Once these patterns are identified, it is important to explore their origins. Self-sabotage often stems from deep-seated beliefs formed through past experiences, societal conditioning, or fear of the unknown. For instance, a belief such as *"I'm not good enough"* might originate from childhood criticism, while *"Success is risky"* could reflect a fear of change or rejection. By uncovering these roots, you gain insight into why self-sabotage occurs and how to address it.

Reframing limiting beliefs is a powerful tool for dismantling self-sabotage. Challenge the narratives that sustain these behaviors by questioning their validity: *Is this belief based on fact or assumption? What evidence contradicts it? How would I act if I believed the opposite?* For example, replacing *"I always fail"* with *"I learn and grow through every experience"* shifts the focus from limitation to possibility.

Another strategy is to set clear and achievable goals. Vague or overly ambitious objectives often trigger self-sabotage, as they create overwhelm or uncertainty. Break larger goals into smaller, manageable steps, celebrating progress along the way. For example, instead of setting a goal to *"write a book,"* start with *"write 500 words a day."* This approach reduces pressure and builds momentum, making it easier to stay on track.

Self-sabotage is often fueled by fear—fear of failure, success, rejection, or the unknown. Addressing these fears directly is essential. Begin by naming the fear and exploring its impact: *What am I afraid will happen? How likely is this outcome? What would I do if it occurred?* Visualization can help reframe fears, imagining yourself navigating challenges successfully and emerging stronger.

Building self-compassion is another key aspect of overcoming self-sabotage. Many self-sabotaging behaviors stem from harsh self-criticism or perfectionism, which create unrealistic expectations and amplify feelings of inadequacy. Practicing self-compassion involves treating yourself with kindness, acknowledging your efforts, and accepting imperfection as part of growth. Affirmations such as *"I am doing my best, and that is enough"* reinforce this mindset, reducing the tendency to sabotage progress.

Accountability provides additional support. Sharing goals with a trusted friend, mentor, or coach creates a sense of responsibility and encouragement. Regular check-ins help track progress, address setbacks, and maintain motivation. For example, partnering with a colleague to review weekly milestones fosters collaboration and reduces the temptation to procrastinate.

Mindfulness also plays a vital role in addressing self-sabotage. By cultivating present-moment awareness, you become more attuned to the thoughts and emotions driving your actions. When self-sabotaging tendencies arise, mindfulness creates a pause, allowing you to choose a different response. For instance, noticing the urge to procrastinate might prompt you to take a single small action instead, breaking the cycle before it gains momentum.

It is important to recognize that overcoming self-sabotage is not about eradicating doubt or fear but about learning to navigate them effectively. Progress may be uneven, with moments of clarity interspersed with setbacks. Approach these setbacks with curiosity rather than judgment, asking: *What triggered this behavior? What can I learn from it? How can I adjust moving forward?* This perspective transforms setbacks into opportunities for growth.

Creating an environment that supports success further reduces the likelihood of self-sabotage. Surround yourself with individuals who inspire and uplift you, and eliminate distractions or triggers that reinforce unhelpful behaviors. For example, organizing your workspace, setting boundaries around social media use, or seeking out a supportive community fosters an atmosphere conducive to focus and progress.

Visualizing success regularly reinforces the mindset and behaviors needed to overcome self-sabotage. Imagine yourself achieving your goals, feeling the emotions associated with accomplishment, and navigating challenges with confidence. This mental rehearsal not only strengthens motivation but also primes the mind to act in alignment with your aspirations.

While the journey to overcoming self-sabotage requires effort and commitment, its rewards are profound. By breaking free from these patterns, you reclaim agency over your choices, aligning your actions with your values and goals. Relationships improve as you engage authentically, and opportunities expand as fear and doubt lose their grip.

Ultimately, self-sabotage is not a reflection of who you are but a signal of where growth is needed. Addressing it with compassion and determination transforms it from a barrier into a bridge, connecting you to your potential and purpose. Through this process, you discover that the greatest ally in your transformation is not an external force but the empowered, self-aware version of yourself waiting to emerge.

In mastering the art of overcoming self-sabotage, you unlock a life of possibility—a life where intentions translate into actions, and dreams evolve into reality. This shift is not merely about eliminating obstacles but about stepping into your power, embracing the fullness of who you are, and creating a future defined by growth, authenticity, and fulfillment.

Chapter 24
Mental Reprogramming

The mind is a complex system of patterns, beliefs, and thought processes that shape how we experience and interact with the world. Over time, these mental frameworks become ingrained, dictating our responses and behaviors, often without conscious awareness. Mental reprogramming is the process of identifying and reshaping these patterns to align with desired outcomes, empowering transformation from within. Using advanced techniques such as those rooted in Neuro-Linguistic Programming (NLP), this practice unlocks the potential to replace limiting thoughts with empowering beliefs.

Mental reprogramming begins with awareness. The mind operates much like a computer, running programs—habits of thought and behavior—on autopilot. These programs are often shaped by early experiences, societal conditioning, or repeated affirmations, both positive and negative. For instance, a person who grew up hearing *"You're not good at math"* may carry an ingrained belief of inadequacy in that area, influencing their confidence and choices long into adulthood. Recognizing these mental scripts is the first step in reprogramming them.

To identify these patterns, start by observing recurring thoughts and behaviors. Journaling can help capture and analyze these patterns, revealing underlying beliefs. For example, frequent thoughts like *"I always fail at this"* or *"Things never work out for me"* point to limiting narratives that need to be addressed. Asking reflective questions such as *"What belief is driving this thought?* or *"Where did this belief originate?"* deepens understanding, transforming unconscious patterns into conscious material for change.

Once limiting beliefs are identified, reframing becomes the next step. Reframing involves challenging the validity of these beliefs and replacing them with empowering alternatives. For example, instead of *"I'm not good at public speaking,"* reframe to *"I am improving my public speaking skills with practice."* This shift acknowledges progress and possibility, dismantling the absolutes that often characterize limiting beliefs.

Visualization is a powerful tool for mental reprogramming. By vividly imagining yourself embodying the desired belief or behavior, you create a mental blueprint for change. For instance, if you aim to replace self-doubt with confidence, visualize yourself successfully navigating a challenging situation, feeling poised and capable. Engage all senses in this visualization—see the environment, hear the supportive words you might say to yourself, and feel the physical sensations of confidence. Repeating this exercise regularly strengthens the neural pathways associated with the new belief.

Affirmations further reinforce mental reprogramming. These are positive, present-tense statements that align with your goals and values. For example, affirming *"I am capable and resilient in the face of challenges"* reconditions the mind to adopt a more empowering narrative. The key to effective affirmations is repetition and emotional engagement; the more you believe and feel the affirmation, the deeper its impact.

Anchoring, a technique from NLP, creates a direct association between a positive state and a physical or sensory trigger. For example, if confidence is the desired state, recall a moment when you felt truly confident, immerse yourself in the memory, and then link it to a physical gesture—such as pressing your thumb and forefinger together. Repeating this process reinforces the association, enabling you to access the confident state on demand.

Mental reprogramming also benefits from mindfulness. Practicing mindfulness helps cultivate a present-focused awareness, reducing the influence of automatic thoughts and reactions. When a limiting belief surfaces, mindfulness allows you to observe it without judgment, creating space to choose a different response. For example, noticing the thought *"I can't handle this"* with mindfulness enables you to pause and consciously reframe it to *"I am learning how to handle this."*

Hypnosis and guided meditation are advanced methods that access the subconscious, where many mental programs reside. During these practices, the mind enters a relaxed state, becoming more receptive to positive suggestions. Listening to guided scripts that align with your goals—such as improving confidence or releasing fear—can accelerate the process of reprogramming, embedding new patterns at a deeper level.

Breaking the cycle of mental patterns also requires consistency and patience. Reprogramming is not an overnight process; it involves repeating new thoughts and behaviors until they become the default. Setbacks are natural and should be met with compassion. Each instance of slipping back into old patterns is an opportunity to practice the new ones, reinforcing progress over time.

An essential component of mental reprogramming is aligning new beliefs with actions. For example, if the reprogrammed belief is *"I am worthy of success,"* act in ways that affirm this belief, such as setting ambitious goals, seeking opportunities, or advocating for yourself in professional settings. These actions create a feedback loop, where behavior reinforces belief and belief reinforces behavior.

Mental reprogramming extends beyond individual transformation; it influences how we interact with others and navigate the world. By adopting empowering beliefs, you radiate confidence, resilience, and positivity, inspiring those around you. For instance, shifting from *"I can't make a difference"* to *"My actions have impact"* not only transforms personal outcomes but also encourages collaborative growth and contribution.

To maintain the benefits of mental reprogramming, regular self-assessment is essential. Periodically revisit your beliefs and goals, ensuring they remain aligned with your evolving aspirations. Life changes, and beliefs that served you in one phase may need adjustment in another. This adaptability ensures that mental reprogramming remains a dynamic and lifelong practice.

Ultimately, mental reprogramming is an act of empowerment. It frees you from the constraints of outdated beliefs, enabling you to create a mindset that supports your vision and values. Through this practice, you reclaim the power to shape your reality, transforming thought into action and potential into achievement.

In mastering mental reprogramming, you discover that the mind is not a fixed entity but a flexible tool, capable of profound transformation. By intentionally reprogramming your mental patterns, you align your thoughts with your goals, unlocking the limitless potential within. This shift is not just a change in perspective; it is a revolution in how you experience and create your life.

Chapter 25
Internal Communication

The dialogues we hold within ourselves shape the way we perceive the world, define our sense of self, and influence our actions. Internal communication, often referred to as self-talk, is the continuous stream of thoughts and narratives that runs through our minds. This inner dialogue can either empower us, fostering growth and resilience, or undermine us, reinforcing doubt and limitation. Cultivating positive and constructive internal communication is a transformative practice, aligning thoughts with intentions and unlocking the path to confidence and self-mastery.

Internal communication begins with awareness. Many people are unaware of the tone and content of their inner dialogue, as it operates on a subconscious level. Yet, the words we say to ourselves carry immense power. For instance, thoughts like *"I always fail"* or *"I'm not good enough"* reinforce a narrative of inadequacy, while affirmations like *"I am learning and improving"* foster self-belief. The first step in reshaping internal communication is observing these patterns without judgment.

Mindfulness practices are invaluable for this awareness. Setting aside moments throughout the day to pause and tune into your thoughts reveals recurring themes and triggers. Journaling provides another method of exploration, capturing internal dialogues in writing for deeper reflection. Ask yourself: *What do I frequently tell myself when I face challenges? How do I speak to myself when I succeed?* These questions illuminate the tone and direction of your self-talk.

Once internal dialogue is recognized, the next step is to evaluate its impact. Does your self-talk motivate and encourage you, or does it create barriers and self-doubt? Negative self-talk often reflects limiting beliefs formed through past experiences or societal conditioning. For example, a critical inner voice might echo past judgments from authority figures or peers. Understanding the origins of these thoughts allows you to approach them with curiosity and compassion rather than resistance.

Reframing is a powerful tool for transforming negative self-talk. This practice involves challenging unhelpful narratives and replacing them with constructive alternatives. For instance, instead of *"I'll never be good at this,"* reframe to *"I'm improving with practice."* Instead of *"I failed,"* try *"I learned something valuable."* Reframing not only shifts perspective but also creates space for growth and resilience.

Affirmations play a central role in fostering positive internal communication. These are intentional, empowering statements that align with your goals and values. Affirmations such as *"I am capable and resourceful"* or *"I trust my ability to navigate challenges"* reinforce confidence and self-worth. The key to effective affirmations is repetition and emotional engagement—saying them with conviction and visualizing their truth strengthens their impact.

Another technique is personifying the inner critic. By giving this critical voice a name or identity, you create distance from its influence. For example, if you label your inner critic "The Doubter," you can respond to it with detachment: *"Thank you for your concern, Doubter, but I'm choosing to focus on what I can achieve."* This practice separates self-worth from the negativity, reducing its hold on your mindset.

Visualization enhances internal communication by creating vivid mental images of success and self-empowerment. Imagine yourself navigating a challenge with confidence, speaking to yourself with kindness and encouragement. Visualize achieving your goals and affirm the steps you are taking to get there. These mental rehearsals reinforce constructive self-talk, embedding it into your subconscious.

Gratitude also transforms internal communication. By focusing on what you appreciate about yourself—your strengths, efforts, and achievements—you shift the narrative from criticism to celebration. For instance, acknowledging your persistence in learning a new skill fosters a sense of pride and motivation. Regularly reflecting on moments of gratitude for yourself strengthens self-compassion, a vital component of healthy internal dialogue.

Boundaries within internal communication are equally important. It is essential to recognize when self-talk becomes overly critical or unrealistic. Setting limits on how much mental energy you devote to certain thoughts prevents them from spiraling into negativity. For example, if you catch yourself ruminating on a mistake, consciously decide to spend only a few minutes reflecting on it before redirecting your focus to solutions or next steps.

Supporting this transformation is the practice of self-compassion. Many people speak to themselves in ways they would never speak to a friend or loved one. Cultivating a kinder, more supportive tone fosters resilience and self-trust. When facing setbacks, replace criticism with understanding: *"It's okay to make mistakes; I'm learning and growing."* This shift from judgment to encouragement builds a foundation of confidence and self-acceptance.

The impact of positive internal communication extends beyond the self. When your inner dialogue aligns with confidence and self-worth, it influences how you engage with others and the world. Relationships benefit as you approach them with authenticity and openness, unburdened by self-doubt. Professional opportunities expand as you communicate with clarity and assurance, reflecting your inner belief in your abilities.

Building effective internal communication is an ongoing process. Like any skill, it requires practice and patience. Setbacks are natural, and moments of negative self-talk will arise. The key is to approach these moments with curiosity rather than frustration, using them as opportunities to reinforce new patterns. Over time, constructive self-talk becomes second nature, guiding you toward greater confidence and fulfillment.

To sustain this practice, create rituals that reinforce positive internal communication. Begin each day with affirmations or a gratitude journal, setting a tone of encouragement and appreciation. Use visualization before tackling challenges, mentally rehearsing success. At the end of the day, reflect on moments where your self-talk supported your growth, celebrating even small victories.

Ultimately, internal communication is the foundation of self-empowerment. It shapes how you perceive yourself, navigate challenges, and pursue your aspirations. By transforming your inner dialogue, you create a mindset that supports your goals and values, fostering a life of authenticity, resilience, and purpose.

In mastering internal communication, you uncover the profound truth that the most important conversations you have are the ones with yourself. Through this practice, you become not only your own advocate but also your greatest ally, unlocking the limitless potential within and shaping a life of empowerment and growth.

Chapter 26
Relaxation Techniques

In the fast-paced rhythms of modern life, stress often takes center stage, affecting the mind, body, and spirit. While challenges are an inevitable part of growth, prolonged tension undermines well-being and limits the ability to think, act, and feel with clarity. Relaxation techniques offer a powerful antidote, providing tools to calm the mind, restore balance, and create a state of receptivity that supports transformation. By cultivating relaxation, we nurture resilience and open pathways for learning, adaptation, and growth.

Relaxation is not simply the absence of stress—it is an active process of resetting the nervous system, allowing the body and mind to shift from a state of heightened alertness to one of calm and restoration. This transition fosters clarity, emotional regulation, and physical recovery, creating the ideal environment for self-transformation.

The practice begins with awareness. Recognizing the signs of stress—whether physical, such as muscle tension or headaches, or emotional, such as irritability or overwhelm—signals the need for relaxation. These cues are the body's way of asking for care, inviting us to pause and recalibrate. By acknowledging these signals without judgment, we take the first step toward managing stress effectively.

Breathing exercises are among the simplest and most effective relaxation techniques. Breath is directly linked to the nervous system, with slow, intentional breathing activating the parasympathetic response—the body's natural state of calm. One popular method is diaphragmatic breathing, which involves inhaling deeply through the nose, allowing the abdomen to expand, and exhaling slowly through the mouth. Another technique, the 4-7-8 method, involves inhaling for four counts, holding the breath for seven counts, and exhaling for eight counts. Both practices create a sense of grounding and ease, even in moments of intense stress.

Progressive muscle relaxation (PMR) is another powerful tool. This technique involves systematically tensing and then releasing different muscle groups, moving from the feet to the head or vice versa. For example, you might clench your fists tightly for a few seconds, then release them fully, noticing the contrast between tension and relaxation. PMR not only reduces physical tension but also enhances mind-body awareness, helping you identify and release areas of stored stress.

Visualization adds a creative dimension to relaxation. By imagining a peaceful scene—a tranquil beach, a quiet forest, or a sunlit meadow—you engage the mind's power to influence the body. Close your eyes and immerse yourself in the details of the scene: the colors, sounds, textures, and sensations. This mental escape creates a sanctuary of calm, interrupting stress and fostering a sense of renewal.

Mindfulness meditation integrates relaxation with present-moment awareness. By focusing on the here and now, mindfulness reduces the mental chatter that often fuels stress. Begin by sitting comfortably and focusing on your breath, observing each inhale and exhale without trying to control them. When your mind wanders, gently bring your attention back to the breath. This practice trains the mind to stay present, cultivating a sense of calm and clarity that carries into daily life.

For those who find movement more conducive to relaxation, practices like yoga or tai chi offer a blend of physical activity and mindfulness. These disciplines emphasize slow, deliberate movements paired with focused breathing, creating a flow state that releases tension and fosters harmony between the mind and body. Even a brief session of gentle stretches can have a profound impact, loosening tight muscles and restoring energy.

Music and sound therapy provide additional pathways to relaxation. Listening to soothing music, nature sounds, or specific frequencies designed for calming the mind can shift your emotional state almost immediately. Some find benefit in binaural beats—audio tracks that use specific tones to induce states of relaxation or focus. Experiment with different sounds to discover what resonates most deeply with you.

Journaling offers a reflective approach to relaxation, providing a space to release thoughts and emotions that might otherwise feel overwhelming. Writing down worries, frustrations, or plans for the future clears mental clutter, creating space for calm. Gratitude journaling, in particular, shifts focus from stressors to positive aspects of life, enhancing emotional resilience.

Creating a relaxation routine ensures these practices become a consistent part of your life. Consider dedicating specific times each day to relaxation, whether in the morning to set a peaceful tone, during a midday break to recharge, or before bed to unwind. Combining multiple techniques—such as starting with deep breathing, followed by visualization, and ending with journaling—maximizes their benefits.

Relaxation also benefits from an intentional environment. Designating a space for relaxation, free from distractions and filled with calming elements like soft lighting, comfortable seating, or pleasant scents, enhances the experience. For instance, lighting a candle or diffusing essential oils like lavender or chamomile creates a sensory cue that signals the mind and body to relax.

It's important to recognize that relaxation is not a one-size-fits-all practice. What works for one person may not work for another. Experimentation is key to discovering the techniques that resonate most deeply with you. The goal is not perfection but consistency—a commitment to prioritizing your well-being through regular moments of calm.

The benefits of relaxation extend far beyond immediate relief. Regular practice enhances emotional regulation, reducing the intensity of reactions to stressors. It improves focus and decision-making, as a calm mind is better equipped to process information and consider options. Physically, relaxation supports immune function, lowers blood pressure, and reduces the risk of stress-related illnesses.

In relationships, relaxation fosters healthier interactions. A calm and centered state allows for more thoughtful responses, greater empathy, and reduced reactivity during conflicts. Professional performance also improves, as relaxation enhances creativity, problem-solving, and resilience in the face of challenges.

Relaxation is not about escaping life's demands but about equipping yourself to meet them with clarity and strength. It is a practice of self-care that acknowledges your inherent worth and the importance of nurturing your inner resources. Through relaxation, you create a foundation of balance and stability that supports every aspect of your transformation journey.

Ultimately, relaxation is an act of reclaiming your power. It reminds you that amidst the noise and chaos of life, there is always a space of calm within—a space you can access at any time. By cultivating this practice, you strengthen your connection to yourself, unlocking the capacity to navigate life's complexities with grace and resilience. In this state of calm, transformation becomes not just possible but inevitable.

Chapter 27
Reframing Trauma

Trauma, whether born from a single moment or a series of events, leaves an indelible mark on the mind, body, and spirit. It often shapes our thoughts, emotions, and behaviors in ways that feel limiting or painful. Yet within the process of healing lies the potential for profound transformation. Reframing trauma is not about erasing its impact or minimizing its significance; it is about shifting the narrative, discovering meaning in adversity, and transforming wounds into wisdom.

Trauma often embeds itself as a story—a narrative that defines our understanding of what happened and how it affects us. These stories are deeply personal, shaped by our perspectives, emotions, and the meaning we assign to the events. For instance, a narrative like *"This happened to me because I'm weak"* perpetuates feelings of shame and powerlessness. Reframing seeks to rewrite these stories, offering a perspective that empowers rather than diminishes.

The first step in reframing trauma is acknowledging its presence. Healing begins with recognizing and validating the impact of the experience. This involves creating a safe space to confront the emotions and memories associated with the trauma, whether through journaling, therapy, or speaking with trusted individuals. The act of naming the experience—*"This happened, and it hurt me deeply"*—is a powerful declaration of truth and a crucial step toward transformation.

Reframing involves shifting focus from the pain of the event to the growth and strength that can emerge from it. This does not mean denying or ignoring the suffering but rather exploring the lessons and insights it reveals. For example, a person who endured a difficult breakup might reframe the experience as an opportunity to rediscover themselves, prioritize self-care, and understand their needs in relationships. Similarly, someone who faced failure in a career venture might view it as a stepping stone to greater resilience and clarity about their goals.

One effective technique for reframing trauma is exploring the narrative through multiple perspectives. Ask yourself: *How might an outsider view this event? What would I say to a friend who went through the same experience? How might I view this differently in five or ten years?* These shifts in perspective help soften the grip of the original narrative, creating space for alternative interpretations.

Visualization supports this process by allowing you to mentally revisit the traumatic event with a sense of agency. Imagine yourself stepping into the past, but this time as the empowered version of yourself—stronger, wiser, and more compassionate. Visualize comforting your past self, offering support and encouragement. This practice not only reframes the memory but also fosters self-compassion, bridging the gap between who you were then and who you are now.

Emotions play a central role in trauma, and reframing involves working through these emotions with care and intention. Suppressing feelings of anger, sadness, or fear only deepens their impact, while acknowledging and expressing them promotes healing. Practices like mindfulness or somatic experiencing, which focus on reconnecting with the body and its sensations, help release emotions stored within the physical self. For example, deep breathing exercises or grounding techniques can bring a sense of safety and calm during moments of emotional overwhelm.

Language is a powerful tool for reframing. The words we use to describe trauma influence how we experience it. Transforming phrases like *"I'm broken because of this"* into *"I am healing from this"* or *"This ruined my life"* into *"This changed my life, and I'm learning to adapt"* shifts the narrative toward growth and recovery. Affirmations that emphasize strength and resilience—*"I am capable of healing"* or *"I am more than what happened to me"*—further reinforce this transformation.

Relationships provide another avenue for reframing trauma. Connecting with others who have faced similar experiences fosters a sense of shared humanity and reduces feelings of isolation. Support groups, therapy sessions, or even candid conversations with trusted friends allow for mutual understanding and validation. Hearing how others have reframed their own trauma can inspire new ways of viewing your journey.

Forgiveness, both of others and oneself, is often a pivotal aspect of reframing. Forgiveness does not excuse harmful actions or invalidate pain; instead, it releases the emotional hold that the trauma has on you. It is an act of reclaiming power, allowing you to move forward without being tethered to resentment or guilt. For example, forgiving someone who hurt you might involve recognizing their flaws or limitations while affirming your boundaries and worth.

Artistic expression offers an alternative pathway to reframing, translating pain into creation. Writing, painting, music, or dance provides a medium to process and reinterpret the trauma. For instance, journaling about the experience can uncover insights, while painting might convey emotions that words cannot capture. These creative acts transform the rawness of trauma into something meaningful and tangible, fostering a sense of agency and renewal.

The practice of gratitude, though challenging in the context of trauma, can also support reframing. Identifying aspects of life that bring comfort, joy, or connection helps shift focus from loss to abundance. For example, reflecting on the support of loved ones during a difficult time highlights the strength of your relationships, offering a counterbalance to the pain.

Reframing trauma is not a linear process, and setbacks are a natural part of the journey. Some memories may feel resistant to change, and moments of regression may arise. Approach these challenges with patience and self-compassion, understanding that healing is a dynamic and ongoing process. Celebrate progress, no matter how small, as each step forward reinforces the path to transformation.

Ultimately, reframing trauma is an act of reclaiming your narrative. It is a declaration that, while you cannot change the past, you can choose how it shapes your future. Through this practice, trauma becomes not a defining wound but a source of strength and insight, revealing the resilience and courage within.

In mastering the art of reframing, you discover that your experiences—no matter how painful—hold the potential for growth and empowerment. This shift is not about erasing the scars but about embracing them as part of your story, a testament to your ability to endure, adapt, and thrive. Through reframing, you transform adversity into a catalyst for a life of authenticity, purpose, and strength.

Chapter 28
Modeling Excellence

Human progress is built on the ability to learn from one another, to observe successful behaviors, and to replicate them in ways that foster personal growth. Modeling excellence is a practice rooted in this principle, drawing inspiration from those who have achieved desired results and adapting their methods to suit one's unique path. Within the framework of Neuro-Linguistic Programming (NLP), modeling excellence becomes a powerful tool for transformation, enabling individuals to bridge the gap between aspiration and achievement.

Excellence, in this context, refers not to perfection but to consistently effective behaviors, skills, and mindsets that lead to success in a particular domain. Whether it is the confidence of a skilled communicator, the discipline of a top athlete, or the creativity of an innovative leader, excellence leaves patterns—repeatable actions and thought processes—that can be identified, studied, and integrated.

The process of modeling begins with clarity. Define the specific qualities or outcomes you wish to achieve. This could be a professional skill, such as public speaking, or a personal attribute, like resilience. For example, if your goal is to become a more effective leader, identify the traits and actions of leaders you admire—confidence, decisiveness, empathy—and focus on understanding how they embody these qualities.

Once the target is clear, the next step is to choose a model—a person who demonstrates excellence in the area you wish to develop. This individual could be a public figure, a mentor, or even a historical figure whose achievements resonate with you. While it is tempting to focus solely on their successes, it is equally important to study how they overcame challenges and setbacks. Excellence is often forged in adversity, and understanding these moments provides a more complete picture.

Observation is central to modeling. Pay close attention to the actions, language, and attitudes of your chosen model. What habits and routines do they maintain? How do they approach problem-solving, decision-making, or interactions with others? If possible, observe them directly—whether in person, through videos, or by studying their written works. For example, analyzing a skilled negotiator's choice of words, tone, and timing can reveal strategies that contribute to their success.

While external behaviors are important, modeling also delves into the internal processes that drive excellence. This includes understanding the model's beliefs, values, and thought patterns. Ask yourself: *What motivates them? What do they believe about themselves, their abilities, or their purpose?* For instance, a successful entrepreneur might hold a belief in the value of perseverance, viewing challenges as opportunities rather than obstacles. Integrating such beliefs into your mindset creates a foundation for similar success.

Language is a key aspect of this internal modeling. Pay attention to the phrases and metaphors your model uses to describe their experiences. These linguistic patterns often reveal how they frame challenges and opportunities. For example, a leader who frequently uses phrases like *"Every problem is a chance to innovate"* demonstrates a mindset of growth and adaptability. Adopting similar language shapes your own perspective, aligning it with the qualities you wish to develop.

Replication involves applying what you have learned from your model to your own life. Start by integrating small, specific actions or habits. For instance, if your model practices a morning routine that includes journaling and goal-setting, experiment with incorporating these practices into your daily life. Over time, these actions become second nature, creating a foundation for further growth.

Adaptation is equally important. While the goal is to emulate excellence, it is not about copying every detail. Instead, tailor the patterns you observe to fit your unique circumstances, strengths, and goals. For example, if your model's approach to time management involves extensive scheduling but you thrive in a more flexible structure, focus on the underlying principle of intentionality and adapt it to your style.

Feedback plays a vital role in refining the modeling process. Regularly assess how well the new behaviors or mindsets are serving you. Are they leading to the desired outcomes? Are there areas where adjustments are needed? Seeking feedback from others—mentors, colleagues, or trusted friends—provides valuable perspectives and helps identify blind spots.

Visualization enhances the practice of modeling. Mentally rehearse yourself embodying the qualities of your chosen model, engaging in their habits and responding to challenges as they would. For example, if you admire a public speaker's poise and presence, visualize yourself speaking with similar confidence, imagining the posture, tone, and energy you would project. This exercise strengthens the neural pathways associated with the desired behaviors, making them more accessible in real life.

Modeling excellence is not limited to individual growth; it also fosters collaboration and innovation. By observing and integrating the strengths of others, you contribute to a culture of learning and adaptability. For example, within a team setting, adopting a colleague's effective communication style might inspire others to do the same, enhancing overall cohesion and productivity.

It is important to recognize that no model is perfect. Everyone, even those we admire most, has flaws and limitations. Approach modeling with a mindset of curiosity and discernment, focusing on the aspects that align with your goals while acknowledging that you are building your own unique path.

As you practice modeling excellence, its impact becomes cumulative. Each habit, mindset, or skill you adopt builds upon the last, creating a ripple effect of growth. Over time, you may find that others begin to look to you as a model, seeking to learn from your journey. This is a testament to the transformative power of the practice, as it not only enhances your own life but also inspires those around you.

Ultimately, modeling excellence is an act of empowerment. It demonstrates that greatness is not reserved for a select few but is accessible to anyone willing to learn, adapt, and grow. By studying and integrating the patterns of those you admire, you unlock your potential to achieve your own version of excellence, one that reflects your values, aspirations, and individuality.

Through this practice, you discover that the path to success is both a personal and collective endeavor, a journey of learning from the best in others to become the best in yourself. In doing so, you not only transform your life but also contribute to a broader legacy of growth, connection, and achievement.

Chapter 29
Internal Alignment

Internal alignment is the harmony between thoughts, emotions, and actions—a state where every aspect of your being works in concert toward a unified purpose. When you are internally aligned, your decisions resonate with your values, your emotions support your goals, and your actions reflect your intentions. This alignment creates a profound sense of authenticity, clarity, and flow, serving as the foundation for sustained personal transformation.

Misalignment, on the other hand, is a common source of frustration and conflict. It occurs when there is a disconnect between your inner world and your outer actions. For example, pursuing a career path that conflicts with your values, suppressing emotions that need acknowledgment, or making decisions that ignore intuition can all lead to feelings of discontent or stagnation. Internal alignment resolves these tensions, fostering coherence and fulfillment.

The process of achieving internal alignment begins with self-awareness. Understanding your core values—the principles that define what matters most to you—is essential. These values act as a compass, guiding decisions and providing a framework for authentic living. Reflect on questions such as: *What truly drives me? What gives my life meaning?* Write down your answers to uncover the themes that anchor your identity and purpose.

Emotions play a crucial role in alignment. They serve as signals, highlighting when something is in harmony or discord with your values. For instance, feelings of excitement or joy often indicate alignment, while frustration or unease may signal a misstep. Cultivating emotional intelligence—the ability to recognize, understand, and manage your emotions—enables you to use these signals effectively. Ask yourself: *What is this emotion telling me? How does it relate to my current situation?*

Mindset is another key component. Limiting beliefs or negative thought patterns often create barriers to alignment. For example, a belief like *"I'm not capable of achieving this"* can undermine your efforts, even if your actions and values are in sync. Identifying and reframing these beliefs—replacing them with empowering alternatives such as *"I am capable of learning and growing"*—supports the alignment process, ensuring that your thoughts reinforce your goals.

Once your values, emotions, and mindset are clear, the next step is to examine your actions. Are they consistent with what you believe and feel? Are you making choices that reflect your authentic self? For example, if you value connection but spend little time nurturing relationships, misalignment may be creating dissatisfaction. Similarly, if you value creativity but neglect opportunities to express it, your actions may not be serving your growth. Aligning actions with values requires intentionality, a commitment to live in accordance with your inner truth.

Alignment also involves integrating intuition—the inner voice that guides decisions beyond logic. Intuition often arises as a gut feeling or subtle knowing, offering insights that may not be immediately explainable. Honoring intuition requires trust and openness, a willingness to listen to your inner wisdom even when external circumstances suggest otherwise. For instance, declining a seemingly lucrative opportunity because it doesn't feel "right" aligns with the integrity of your intuition.

Conflict often arises when different aspects of yourself pull in opposing directions. For example, a desire for financial stability might conflict with a yearning for creative freedom, or a sense of duty might clash with personal aspirations. Resolving these conflicts requires dialogue with yourself—exploring each perspective with curiosity and compassion. Ask questions like: *What does each part of me need? How can I honor these needs without compromising my values?* Finding a middle ground often reveals solutions that balance competing priorities.

Visualization is a powerful tool for cultivating internal alignment. Imagine yourself living a fully aligned life, where every decision, emotion, and action reflects your values and goals. What does this look like? How does it feel? Engaging in this mental rehearsal creates a blueprint for alignment, reinforcing the connections between your inner and outer worlds.

Journaling further supports this process. Regularly reflecting on your experiences, decisions, and emotions provides insights into where alignment exists and where adjustments are needed. Use prompts such as: *When did I feel most at peace this week? What actions felt disconnected from my values? What small change can I make today to move closer to alignment?*

Boundaries are another critical aspect of internal alignment. Misalignment often occurs when you prioritize external demands over internal needs. Setting and maintaining boundaries ensures that your time, energy, and focus remain aligned with your priorities. For example, saying no to commitments that drain you or create conflict with your values preserves space for what truly matters.

Building internal alignment is an ongoing process, one that requires patience and adaptability. Life's complexities often introduce new challenges or shifts in priorities, and alignment must evolve to reflect these changes. Periodically reassessing your values, goals, and actions ensures that you remain on a path of authenticity and growth.

The benefits of internal alignment are profound. It fosters a sense of peace and confidence, as your actions no longer feel at odds with your intentions. Decisions become clearer, guided by the integrity of your values and emotions. Relationships deepen, as authenticity strengthens connections with others. Challenges, rather than derailing progress, become opportunities to reaffirm your alignment and resilience.

In professional contexts, internal alignment enhances effectiveness and fulfillment. When your work aligns with your values and goals, you approach tasks with greater enthusiasm and purpose. For instance, aligning a career in environmental advocacy with a value of sustainability creates a sense of meaning and impact, driving both personal and professional satisfaction.

Ultimately, internal alignment is the foundation of a life well-lived. It transforms the fragmented experience of disconnection into a cohesive journey of authenticity and purpose. Through this practice, you create a harmonious relationship with yourself, one where every thought, feeling, and action contributes to your highest aspirations.

In mastering internal alignment, you discover that true transformation arises not from external circumstances but from the coherence of your inner world. This harmony empowers you to navigate life with clarity, resilience, and joy, building a future that reflects the fullest expression of who you are.

Chapter 30
Mental Resilience

Mental resilience is the capacity to navigate life's challenges with strength, adaptability, and purpose. It is not about avoiding hardship but about thriving in the face of adversity, using difficulties as opportunities for growth. Building resilience strengthens your ability to recover from setbacks, maintain focus under pressure, and remain true to your goals despite life's uncertainties. It is an essential skill in personal transformation, empowering you to sustain progress and cultivate a sense of inner stability.

At its core, mental resilience begins with mindset. How you perceive challenges shapes your ability to confront them. Viewing obstacles as opportunities rather than insurmountable barriers creates a foundation for resilience. This shift involves reframing setbacks as lessons, asking: *What can I learn from this experience? How can I grow through it?* For example, a failed project might reveal areas for improvement or spark innovation, transforming disappointment into motivation.

Self-awareness is a cornerstone of resilience. Understanding your emotional and mental responses to stress provides clarity on how to navigate difficulties effectively. This requires observing your reactions without judgment, identifying triggers, and recognizing patterns that may undermine your resilience. For instance, noticing that self-doubt arises during high-stakes situations allows you to prepare strategies for managing it, such as affirmations or grounding techniques.

Stress management is another key aspect of resilience. Chronic stress depletes mental resources, making it harder to adapt and recover. Techniques such as mindfulness meditation, deep breathing, or progressive muscle relaxation help regulate the body's stress response, creating a calm and focused state. For example, practicing diaphragmatic breathing during moments of tension can reduce anxiety and restore clarity, allowing you to approach challenges with a steady mind.

Cultivating a growth mindset is essential for resilience. This mindset embraces the belief that abilities and intelligence can develop through effort and learning. When setbacks occur, a growth mindset focuses on what can be improved rather than dwelling on failure. For instance, instead of thinking *"I'm not good at this,"* a growth mindset reframes to *"I'm learning and improving with practice."* This perspective fosters persistence and adaptability, both critical components of resilience.

Building resilience also involves setting realistic expectations. Perfectionism—expecting flawless outcomes in every situation—often undermines resilience by amplifying self-criticism and fear of failure. Embracing imperfection as a natural part of growth reduces pressure and encourages experimentation. For instance, approaching a new skill with the mindset of *"I'll do my best and learn along the way"* creates space for both success and mistakes, fostering resilience through experience.

Connection plays a vital role in resilience. Supportive relationships provide emotional strength, perspective, and encouragement during difficult times. Cultivating a network of trusted friends, mentors, or colleagues creates a foundation of mutual support, where challenges are shared, and solutions are co-created. For example, discussing a career setback with a mentor might reveal insights or opportunities that you hadn't considered, helping you move forward.

Resilience is also strengthened by practicing gratitude. Reflecting on the positive aspects of your life, even amidst hardship, shifts focus from scarcity to abundance. For instance, during a period of financial stress, gratitude for supportive relationships or personal health reminds you of the resources and strengths already present in your life. This practice nurtures optimism and reinforces the belief that challenges can be overcome.

Adaptability is another hallmark of resilience. Life's unpredictability requires flexibility, the ability to adjust plans and expectations when circumstances change. This might involve reevaluating goals, exploring alternative solutions, or accepting temporary setbacks while maintaining a long-term vision. For example, pivoting to a new strategy after an unexpected challenge at work demonstrates adaptability and keeps progress on track.

Physical well-being supports mental resilience. The mind and body are deeply interconnected, and maintaining physical health enhances your capacity to handle stress and adversity. Regular exercise, a balanced diet, and sufficient sleep create a foundation of energy and vitality, strengthening resilience from the inside out. For instance, a brisk walk or a yoga session can clear the mind, boost mood, and improve focus, all of which contribute to a resilient mindset.

Resilience also involves cultivating hope and optimism. These qualities do not ignore challenges but emphasize the possibility of positive outcomes. Visualizing success, focusing on strengths, and affirming your ability to overcome difficulties foster a sense of agency and confidence. For example, imagining yourself achieving a goal despite setbacks reinforces the belief that progress is possible, even in the face of obstacles.

Practical tools enhance resilience in daily life. Journaling provides a structured way to process emotions, reflect on experiences, and identify solutions. Writing about challenges, alongside the steps you've taken to address them, reinforces a sense of progress and capability. Similarly, affirmations such as *"I am strong, adaptable, and capable of overcoming challenges"* serve as daily reminders of your resilience.

Resilience is not a fixed trait but a skill that grows with intention and effort. Setbacks and struggles are natural parts of life, and moments of vulnerability do not diminish your strength. Instead, they highlight areas for growth, inviting you to deepen your resilience through reflection and action. Each time you recover from difficulty, your capacity for resilience expands, equipping you for future challenges.

The benefits of resilience extend beyond handling adversity. A resilient mindset fosters creativity, problem-solving, and emotional stability, enhancing your ability to thrive in all areas of life. Relationships benefit from the patience and understanding that resilience cultivates, while professional endeavors gain from your ability to navigate complexity and uncertainty with confidence.

Ultimately, mental resilience is the art of rising—not only from setbacks but also into your potential. It empowers you to face life's challenges with courage and clarity, transforming obstacles into stepping stones for growth. Through this practice, you discover that resilience is not merely a response to difficulty but a pathway to mastery, a testament to the strength and adaptability within you.

In building mental resilience, you cultivate a foundation of inner strength that supports every aspect of your transformation journey. This strength, rooted in self-awareness, adaptability, and hope, becomes your anchor in the ever-changing tides of life, guiding you toward a future defined by growth, purpose, and possibility.

Chapter 31
Breaking Limits

Limits are often self-imposed, shaped by beliefs, experiences, and societal expectations that create invisible boundaries around what we think we can achieve. While these limits may feel real, they are often constructs of the mind, rooted in fear, doubt, or habit. Breaking limits is the process of recognizing, challenging, and expanding these boundaries, allowing you to step into your fullest potential. It is a journey of courage and self-discovery, transforming limitations into opportunities for growth.

The first step in breaking limits is identifying them. This requires honest introspection and awareness of the beliefs and patterns that constrain you. These limits often appear as internal statements: *"I could never do that," "I'm not good enough,"* or *"That's just not possible for me."* Journaling is a valuable tool for uncovering these thoughts, providing a space to explore where and how they arise. Ask yourself: *What do I avoid because I think I can't succeed? What assumptions do I make about my abilities or potential?*

Once identified, the origins of these limits often reveal themselves. Many are rooted in past experiences—moments of failure, rejection, or criticism—that left an imprint on your self-perception. Others may stem from societal norms or external expectations that subtly dictate what is deemed possible or acceptable. Recognizing these origins allows you to approach your limits with understanding and compassion, rather than judgment or frustration.

Challenging these limits involves questioning their validity. Are they based on evidence, or are they assumptions? For instance, a belief like *"I'm terrible at public speaking"* might stem from a single uncomfortable experience, but it does not define your future capabilities. Reframing these beliefs—shifting from *"I can't"* to *"I'm learning"*—creates space for growth. Affirmations such as *"I am capable of improving with effort and practice"* reinforce this new narrative.

Expanding the comfort zone is a crucial aspect of breaking limits. Comfort zones, while safe and familiar, often act as barriers to growth. Stepping beyond them requires intentionality and small, manageable steps. For example, if networking feels intimidating, start by attending a casual gathering or initiating one-on-one conversations before progressing to larger events. Each step builds confidence, proving to yourself that the boundaries you perceived are not fixed.

Visualization is a powerful tool in this process. Imagine yourself successfully achieving what once felt impossible, engaging all your senses to make the experience vivid and real. For instance, if you aim to run a marathon but feel limited by doubt, visualize yourself crossing the finish line, feeling strong and accomplished. This mental rehearsal not only boosts confidence but also primes the mind for action, bridging the gap between imagination and reality.

Facing fear is integral to breaking limits. Fear often signals the edge of the comfort zone, a boundary that, once crossed, leads to growth. Instead of avoiding fear, approach it with curiosity: *What is this fear trying to protect me from? What might I gain by moving through it?* Techniques such as deep breathing, mindfulness, or reframing fear as excitement can help manage its intensity, allowing you to act despite it.

Support from others accelerates the process of breaking limits. Mentors, coaches, or supportive friends can provide perspective, encouragement, and accountability. They may see potential in you that you cannot yet recognize in yourself, offering guidance and reassurance as you navigate new challenges. Sharing your goals with others also reinforces commitment, as accountability adds an external layer of motivation.

Breaking limits often involves experimentation and failure. Embracing failure as a natural part of growth is essential. Each misstep offers valuable lessons, revealing areas for improvement and resilience. For instance, an entrepreneur facing setbacks in a new business venture might gain insights into market demands, financial management, or personal strengths. Reframing failure as feedback transforms it from a deterrent into a catalyst for progress.

Celebrating small victories along the way reinforces momentum and motivation. Each achievement, no matter how minor, proves that limits can be expanded. For example, if you previously avoided speaking up in meetings, successfully contributing once is a milestone worth acknowledging. These celebrations create positive reinforcement, encouraging continued effort.

As you break through one limit, new ones often appear. This is a natural part of growth, as the boundaries of possibility expand with each success. Approaching these new challenges with the same mindset of curiosity and courage ensures that growth remains continuous. Regular reflection—through journaling, meditation, or discussions with trusted individuals—helps track progress and identify new areas for exploration.

The benefits of breaking limits extend far beyond the immediate achievement of goals. Each boundary crossed strengthens confidence, resilience, and self-belief, creating a ripple effect across all areas of life. Relationships deepen as you engage with others authentically, unburdened by self-doubt. Professional opportunities expand as you take on challenges with assurance and creativity. Most importantly, breaking limits fosters a profound sense of freedom, as you realize that many constraints are self-imposed and therefore within your power to change.

Ultimately, breaking limits is not just about surpassing what you once thought possible—it is about redefining who you are and what you are capable of. It is an act of liberation, a declaration that you will not be confined by fear, doubt, or convention. Through this process, you transform limitations into stepping stones, building a life of purpose, growth, and fulfillment.

In mastering the art of breaking limits, you discover that the boundaries of possibility are far wider than you imagined. Each step beyond a perceived limit reaffirms the truth that you are capable of more than you believed, empowering you to live with authenticity, courage, and boundless potential.

Chapter 32
Body Language

The way we move, gesture, and hold ourselves speaks volumes, often revealing more than words can convey. Body language is a powerful form of nonverbal communication, shaping how we interact with others and how we perceive ourselves. It reflects emotional states, confidence levels, and intentions, influencing both interpersonal dynamics and internal experiences. Understanding and consciously using body language can transform how you communicate, connect, and carry yourself, becoming a cornerstone of personal transformation.

Body language operates on two levels: outwardly, in how others interpret your gestures and posture, and inwardly, in how it affects your emotions and mindset. For example, standing tall with an open posture conveys confidence and approachability, both to others and to yourself. Conversely, slouching or crossing your arms might signal defensiveness or discomfort, even if unintended.

Awareness is the first step in harnessing the power of body language. Begin by observing your habitual movements, postures, and gestures throughout the day. How do you stand, sit, or walk? What signals might you be sending in conversations or meetings? Journaling about your observations or asking for feedback from trusted friends or colleagues can provide valuable insights into your nonverbal patterns.

Posture is a foundational element of body language. An aligned and upright posture not only projects confidence but also supports physical well-being. Imagine a string gently pulling the crown of your head upward, elongating your spine while keeping your shoulders relaxed. This simple adjustment creates an air of self-assurance and openness, inviting positive interactions and feelings of empowerment.

Facial expressions are equally significant. The face often serves as the primary focus in communication, expressing emotions such as joy, concern, or curiosity. Practicing mindful awareness of your expressions—such as softening your gaze, maintaining eye contact, or offering a genuine smile—enhances rapport and trust. For instance, in a professional setting, nodding while listening conveys engagement and attentiveness, strengthening the connection with your audience.

Gestures add emphasis and clarity to verbal communication. Open gestures, such as extending your hands with palms visible, signal honesty and inclusivity. On the other hand, closed or erratic gestures can create confusion or unease. Practicing intentional gestures, aligned with your words and tone, reinforces your message and ensures that your body language supports rather than detracts from your communication.

Mirroring is a subtle yet effective technique for building rapport. By reflecting the body language of the person you are interacting with—such as matching their posture or pace of movement—you create a sense of connection and understanding. For example, if someone leans slightly forward during a conversation, doing the same conveys alignment and attentiveness. However, mirroring should be natural and understated to avoid appearing forced or insincere.

The concept of power poses demonstrates the inward impact of body language. Research suggests that expansive poses—such as standing with your feet shoulder-width apart and hands on your hips—can increase feelings of confidence and reduce stress. Incorporating such poses into your routine, even for a few minutes before a challenging task, primes your mindset for success. For instance, adopting a power pose before a presentation helps shift your energy toward assurance and composure.

Body language is also deeply connected to emotional regulation. Certain movements or gestures can help release tension, calm anxiety, or enhance focus. For example, taking slow, deliberate breaths while rolling your shoulders backward can ease physical and emotional stress, creating a sense of relaxation. Grounding techniques, such as planting your feet firmly on the floor and centering your posture, anchor you in the present moment, reducing feelings of overwhelm.

Cultural awareness is essential when interpreting and using body language. Gestures and postures that convey one meaning in one culture may carry a different or even opposite meaning in another. For example, maintaining prolonged eye contact might signal confidence in some cultures but be considered intrusive in others. Sensitivity to these nuances ensures that your body language remains respectful and effective in diverse contexts.

Body language also influences self-perception. Adopting positive and intentional body language shapes not only how others see you but also how you see yourself. For instance, practicing a confident stance regularly reinforces a sense of self-assuredness over time. This feedback loop between body and mind becomes a powerful tool for personal growth and transformation.

Practical exercises can help integrate intentional body language into daily life. Start by practicing in front of a mirror, observing how adjustments in posture, facial expressions, or gestures change your appearance and energy. Record yourself speaking, noting how your body language aligns with or detracts from your message. Over time, these practices build awareness and refine your ability to communicate effectively.

Nonverbal cues also play a pivotal role in relationships. Attuning to the body language of others allows you to respond with empathy and understanding, deepening connections. For example, noticing when someone's posture tightens or gaze shifts might indicate discomfort, prompting you to adjust your approach or offer reassurance. Similarly, mirroring positive cues like a smile or nod fosters trust and alignment.

Balancing congruence between verbal and nonverbal communication is essential. Mismatched signals—for instance, saying *"I'm excited"* while displaying a neutral or closed posture—can create confusion or doubt. Striving for consistency between words and body language ensures that your message resonates clearly and authentically.

Over time, the conscious use of body language becomes second nature, enhancing your presence and influence in all areas of life. It complements verbal communication, creating a holistic and impactful expression of your thoughts, emotions, and intentions. Whether navigating professional interactions, deepening personal relationships, or building confidence, body language serves as a silent yet powerful ally.

Ultimately, mastering body language is about alignment—between your inner state and your outward expression. By cultivating awareness and intention, you unlock the potential to communicate with clarity, authenticity, and purpose. Through this practice, you not only transform how others perceive you but also strengthen your connection to yourself, creating a foundation for lasting growth and fulfillment.

In mastering the language of the body, you discover that transformation is not just about words or actions but about how you embody your truth. Each gesture, posture, and movement becomes a reflection of your inner strength, empowering you to engage with the world with confidence and grace.

Chapter 33
The Cycle of Change

Change is the essence of growth, a natural rhythm that governs both life and personal transformation. Yet, the process of change is often met with resistance, uncertainty, and emotional upheaval. The cycle of change provides a framework for understanding the stages we navigate as we adapt, evolve, and create new realities. By recognizing these stages and learning to work with them, we can approach transformation with clarity, resilience, and purpose.

The cycle of change is not a linear path but a dynamic process that unfolds in stages. Each stage carries its own challenges and opportunities, contributing to the overall journey of transformation. While the specifics of these stages may vary, the following core phases often define the process: Awareness, Resistance, Exploration, Action, and Integration.

Awareness is the first stage, where the need or desire for change becomes evident. This awareness may arise from dissatisfaction, a longing for growth, or external circumstances that disrupt the status quo. For example, noticing a lack of fulfillment in a career might spark the realization that change is necessary. This stage often brings mixed emotions—hope for something new and fear of leaving the familiar. Embracing this awareness with curiosity rather than judgment sets the stage for transformation.

Resistance often follows awareness. This stage is marked by reluctance, self-doubt, or fear, as the mind clings to the comfort of the known. Resistance might manifest as procrastination, rationalization, or heightened anxiety. For instance, someone aware of the need to adopt healthier habits might resist by focusing on perceived barriers, such as lack of time or resources. Recognizing resistance as a natural part of change helps reframe it as a protective mechanism rather than a failure. Techniques such as journaling about fears or discussing them with a trusted confidant can help navigate this stage.

The next phase, **Exploration**, involves actively seeking possibilities and envisioning new paths. This stage is characterized by curiosity and experimentation. For example, someone exploring career change might research industries, attend networking events, or take a course to develop new skills. This phase often requires flexibility, as not every avenue will lead to success. The key is to remain open to discovery, allowing the process to refine and clarify your direction.

Action is the turning point in the cycle of change, where intentions solidify into tangible steps. This stage demands commitment, focus, and persistence. Actions may be small, such as updating a résumé or setting aside time for a new hobby, or significant, such as moving to a new city or launching a project. While this phase is energizing, it also requires resilience, as setbacks and challenges often arise. Celebrating progress, no matter how minor, reinforces momentum and strengthens confidence.

The final stage, **Integration**, involves internalizing the changes made and weaving them into your identity and daily life. This is where transformation becomes sustainable, as new behaviors, beliefs, and patterns take root. For instance, someone who has embraced mindfulness practices might find them naturally integrated into their routine, fostering long-term well-being. Reflecting on the journey—what has been learned, gained, and let go—brings closure to this cycle, preparing you for future growth.

It is important to recognize that the cycle of change is iterative. Life continuously presents new opportunities and challenges, and each completed cycle prepares you for the next. For example, mastering one aspect of personal growth, such as improving communication skills, often reveals other areas for development, such as enhancing emotional intelligence. Viewing change as an ongoing journey rather than a destination fosters adaptability and resilience.

Emotions play a central role in the cycle of change. Each stage brings its own emotional landscape—excitement during exploration, frustration during resistance, or pride during integration. Acknowledging and processing these emotions is crucial. Practices such as mindfulness, journaling, or speaking with a supportive friend or coach provide outlets for navigating the emotional complexities of change.

Support systems are invaluable throughout the cycle. Surrounding yourself with individuals who encourage and inspire you creates a foundation of accountability and strength. Whether through mentors, peer groups, or loved ones, their insights and encouragement often illuminate possibilities and pathways that might otherwise go unnoticed.

Breaking the cycle into manageable steps reduces overwhelm. Large goals can feel daunting, but dividing them into smaller, actionable tasks makes progress more achievable. For instance, someone aiming to write a book might start with a daily goal of 500 words, gradually building toward the larger vision. Each completed step reinforces the belief that change is possible.

While the cycle of change offers structure, it is not rigid. Life is unpredictable, and progress may involve detours, pauses, or regressions. These moments are not failures but opportunities to recalibrate and reassess. For example, if resistance resurfaces during the action phase, revisiting the exploration stage to gather more information or refine your approach can reignite momentum.

Visualization enhances the process of change by connecting you with the desired outcome. Picture yourself successfully navigating each stage, from embracing awareness to celebrating integration. Engage all your senses, imagining the emotions, sights, and experiences associated with your transformed self. This mental rehearsal strengthens motivation and clarity, anchoring your efforts in a vivid and compelling vision.

The benefits of embracing the cycle of change are transformative. It fosters self-awareness, resilience, and adaptability, equipping you to navigate life's uncertainties with confidence. Relationships deepen as you engage with others authentically, unafraid to embrace growth. Professionally, the ability to adapt and innovate enhances opportunities and impact. Most importantly, the cycle of change empowers you to live intentionally, shaping your life in alignment with your values and aspirations.

Ultimately, the cycle of change is a journey of becoming—a process of shedding old layers and stepping into new possibilities. By understanding and embracing this cycle, you unlock the power to transform challenges into stepping stones, creating a life defined by growth, purpose, and fulfillment.

Through the practice of navigating change, you discover that transformation is not a single event but a continuous unfolding. Each cycle builds upon the last, revealing deeper insights, greater strengths, and new horizons. In mastering the art of change, you embrace the truth that growth is not only possible but limitless.

Chapter 34
The Power of Feedback

Feedback is a mirror that reflects our actions, behaviors, and impact on others, offering invaluable insights for growth and transformation. It is both a gift and a tool—a way to refine our efforts, deepen self-awareness, and foster connections with others. Mastering the art of giving and receiving feedback empowers us to navigate challenges, strengthen relationships, and continuously improve.

At its essence, feedback provides information about the gap between intention and perception. For example, a leader who believes they are approachable might learn through feedback that team members hesitate to share concerns, highlighting areas for improvement. Embracing feedback with openness allows us to bridge such gaps, aligning our actions with our intentions.

Receiving feedback begins with a mindset of curiosity and willingness. It requires setting aside defensiveness and viewing feedback as an opportunity rather than a critique. This perspective transforms potentially uncomfortable conversations into moments of learning and growth. Ask yourself: *What can I learn from this? How can I use this insight to improve?* Approaching feedback with this attitude fosters resilience and adaptability.

The way feedback is delivered significantly influences how it is received. Constructive feedback is specific, actionable, and rooted in care. For instance, instead of saying *"You're not a good listener,"* constructive feedback might be: *"During meetings, I notice you sometimes interrupt before others finish speaking. Pausing before responding might help everyone feel heard."* This approach focuses on behaviors rather than personal traits, making the feedback easier to process and apply.

When receiving feedback, active listening is crucial. Resist the urge to interrupt, justify, or dismiss what is being shared. Instead, focus on understanding the feedback fully. Reflective responses—such as *"If I understand correctly, you're suggesting I could improve by..."*—demonstrate engagement and ensure clarity. Even if the feedback feels challenging, acknowledging its value fosters mutual respect and trust.

Emotionally, feedback can be complex, particularly when it touches on sensitive areas. Practicing mindfulness during these moments helps regulate emotional responses, creating space to process the information constructively. Techniques like deep breathing or pausing before responding allow you to navigate feedback with composure, maintaining a focus on growth rather than defensiveness.

Not all feedback will resonate, and discernment is essential. Consider the source, context, and intent behind the feedback. For instance, feedback from a trusted mentor about a recurring behavior may carry more weight than a passing comment from an unfamiliar acquaintance. Evaluate the feedback objectively, asking: *Does this align with my goals? Is there truth in this perspective, even if it feels uncomfortable?* Extracting value from feedback, even when it is imperfect, demonstrates emotional intelligence and adaptability.

Seeking feedback proactively enhances personal and professional development. Regularly inviting input from colleagues, friends, or mentors signals a commitment to growth and fosters an open, collaborative environment. For example, asking a colleague, *"What's one thing I could do differently to improve our collaboration?"* invites constructive dialogue and strengthens relationships. Consistent feedback-seeking also reduces the stigma or tension often associated with unsolicited criticism.

Giving feedback effectively is equally important. Begin with a clear intention—feedback should aim to support, guide, or inspire improvement, never to criticize or demean. Start by highlighting strengths before addressing areas for growth, a technique often referred to as the "feedback sandwich." For example: *"You handled the client presentation with confidence and clarity. One area to refine might be including more visual examples to enhance engagement. Overall, your delivery was very strong."* This balance of encouragement and constructive insight creates a positive and actionable message.

Timing matters when delivering feedback. Offering input immediately after an event ensures relevance and clarity, while waiting too long risks diluting its impact. However, it's equally important to choose a moment when both parties are receptive. Providing feedback during a heated moment or when emotions are high may hinder effective communication. Instead, opt for a calm, private setting that fosters dialogue and understanding.

Nonverbal communication plays a significant role in feedback exchanges. Maintaining open body language, making eye contact, and using a warm tone reinforce the intention of care and support. Conversely, crossed arms, avoidance of eye contact, or a harsh tone may unintentionally create barriers, even if the feedback itself is constructive.

Feedback also thrives in an environment of trust and mutual respect. Building a culture of openness—whether in personal relationships, workplaces, or teams—encourages honest and constructive exchanges. For instance, leaders who model vulnerability by seeking feedback from their teams create a ripple effect, inspiring others to do the same. This openness fosters collaboration and continuous improvement.

Reflecting on feedback received and given enhances its value. After receiving feedback, take time to process it, identifying actionable steps and integrating them into your efforts. Similarly, after offering feedback, reflect on the response: *Did my message resonate? Was it delivered in a way that encouraged growth?* These reflections refine your feedback skills, making future exchanges more effective.

Feedback is not only a tool for individual growth but also a driver of collective success. In team settings, constructive feedback fosters innovation, problem-solving, and trust. For example, in a brainstorming session, encouraging diverse perspectives and providing constructive input on ideas strengthens outcomes and builds a sense of shared ownership.

It's important to recognize that feedback is not always easy, especially when addressing deeply ingrained habits or behaviors. Patience and persistence are key. Growth takes time, and incremental progress should be celebrated. For instance, if feedback about time management leads to small but consistent improvements, acknowledge these steps as milestones on the journey to mastery.

Ultimately, the power of feedback lies in its ability to transform potential into reality. It illuminates blind spots, challenges comfort zones, and unlocks opportunities for growth that might otherwise go unnoticed. Embracing feedback as an integral part of transformation shifts it from a source of discomfort to a catalyst for change.

In mastering the art of feedback, you cultivate a mindset of continuous learning and collaboration. You discover that growth is not a solitary endeavor but a shared process, enriched by the insights and perspectives of others. Through feedback, you not only elevate your own potential but also contribute to a culture of mutual support, empowerment, and collective success.

Chapter 35
Emotions as Guides

Emotions are powerful messengers, revealing our deepest needs, desires, and fears. They serve as a compass, guiding us toward growth and transformation. While emotions are often misunderstood or suppressed, learning to interpret and harness them is essential for living authentically and effectively. Embracing emotions as guides unlocks their potential to inform decisions, strengthen relationships, and inspire personal evolution.

At their core, emotions are signals. They arise in response to internal or external events, providing insight into how a situation aligns with our values, goals, and well-being. For example, joy signals alignment and fulfillment, while anger may highlight a perceived injustice or boundary violation. Understanding these signals transforms emotions from obstacles into allies, empowering us to act with clarity and purpose.

The first step in using emotions as guides is awareness. Many people experience emotions as fleeting or overwhelming sensations without pausing to reflect on their origins or meanings. Cultivating mindfulness allows us to observe emotions as they arise, creating space to explore their messages. Ask yourself: *What am I feeling right now? What triggered this emotion? What is it trying to tell me?* These questions deepen self-awareness and encourage constructive engagement with emotions.

Journaling provides a structured way to explore emotions. Writing about your feelings and their associated thoughts or events clarifies patterns and insights. For example, if frustration frequently arises during specific interactions, journaling might reveal unmet needs or misaligned expectations. This practice turns emotions into valuable data, informing decisions and actions.

Emotions are often categorized as "positive" or "negative," but this binary perspective limits their potential. Every emotion, even those we perceive as uncomfortable, carries important information. Sadness, for instance, may signal a need for rest or reflection, while fear might highlight areas requiring preparation or caution. By reframing emotions as neither good nor bad but as meaningful, we create an open, nonjudgmental relationship with them.

Processing emotions effectively is key to harnessing their guidance. Suppressing emotions can lead to physical tension, stress, or emotional outbursts, while overidentifying with emotions can cloud judgment. Practices such as deep breathing, grounding techniques, or somatic awareness help regulate emotions, allowing us to respond rather than react. For instance, taking a moment to breathe deeply during anger creates the space needed to address its underlying cause constructively.

Each emotion offers specific guidance. Joy, for example, illuminates what brings meaning and satisfaction. Paying attention to joyful moments helps clarify passions and priorities, guiding you toward a more fulfilling life. Gratitude amplifies this effect, shifting focus to abundance and strengthening resilience. Incorporating a daily gratitude practice—such as listing three things you appreciate—reinforces positive emotional patterns.

Anger, often misunderstood, serves as a signal that something important needs attention. It may point to boundary violations, unmet needs, or a sense of injustice. Rather than suppressing anger, explore its root cause: *What triggered this emotion? What action can I take to address it constructively?* For example, if anger arises during a disagreement, it might reveal a need for clearer communication or mutual understanding.

Fear, while frequently avoided, is a guide to growth. It often marks the edge of the comfort zone, signaling opportunities for learning and transformation. By approaching fear with curiosity rather than avoidance, you uncover its message: *What am I afraid of? What is this fear protecting me from? What might I gain by moving through it?* For instance, fear of public speaking might point to a desire for greater confidence and self-expression, inspiring steps toward mastery.

Sadness encourages introspection and healing. It invites us to slow down, reflect, and release what no longer serves us. Allowing yourself to feel sadness without judgment creates a space for processing loss or change, fostering emotional resilience. Practices like journaling, talking with a trusted friend, or engaging in creative expression support this process, transforming sadness into insight.

Even emotions like jealousy or envy carry valuable guidance. These emotions often highlight unmet desires or aspirations. For example, feeling envious of a colleague's promotion might reveal your own career ambitions, prompting you to set goals or seek opportunities for growth. By examining these emotions with honesty, you uncover hidden motivations and clarify your path forward.

The body plays a crucial role in emotional awareness. Emotions are not just mental phenomena—they are experienced physically. Tension in the shoulders, a racing heart, or a sinking feeling in the stomach all provide clues to our emotional state. Reconnecting with the body through practices like yoga, tai chi, or mindful movement enhances emotional intelligence, helping you identify and address emotions before they escalate.

Relationships thrive when emotions are used as guides. Sharing your feelings openly and authentically fosters connection and trust. For example, expressing vulnerability—*"I feel hurt because I value our relationship and want to resolve this issue"*— invites understanding and collaboration. Similarly, attuning to the emotions of others deepens empathy, allowing you to respond with care and support.

Boundaries play a vital role in emotional guidance. Emotions often signal when boundaries need to be set or reinforced. For instance, recurring feelings of exhaustion or resentment might indicate overcommitment, prompting a need to prioritize self-care. Honoring these signals strengthens your ability to protect your energy and well-being, enhancing emotional balance.

Over time, using emotions as guides becomes a natural and intuitive practice. Regular reflection—through journaling, mindfulness, or conversation—integrates emotional insights into daily life, enriching decision-making and self-awareness. By honoring emotions rather than resisting or suppressing them, you create a harmonious relationship with yourself, fostering growth and authenticity.

The benefits of embracing emotions as guides extend far beyond personal transformation. Professionally, emotional intelligence enhances communication, leadership, and teamwork, creating environments of collaboration and trust. In relationships, understanding and expressing emotions deepen connection and mutual respect. Most importantly, using emotions as guides aligns your inner world with your outer actions, creating a life of integrity and purpose.

Ultimately, emotions are not obstacles to overcome but allies to embrace. They are the language of the soul, pointing the way toward healing, growth, and fulfillment. By listening to their messages and acting on their guidance, you unlock the wisdom within, transforming every emotion into a step toward your highest potential.

In mastering the art of using emotions as guides, you discover that transformation begins within. Each feeling, no matter how fleeting or intense, carries the seeds of insight and empowerment. By cultivating a relationship of trust and openness with your emotions, you navigate life with authenticity, courage, and grace, creating a future shaped by clarity and intention.

Chapter 36
Habit Transformation

Habits are the invisible architecture of our lives, shaping our daily actions and long-term outcomes. They are routines and behaviors that operate automatically, often without conscious thought. While some habits support growth and well-being, others act as barriers, reinforcing limitations or draining energy. Habit transformation is the process of reshaping these patterns to align with your goals, values, and aspirations. It is a deliberate and empowering practice, enabling sustained progress and personal evolution.

The cycle of habit formation begins with a trigger—a cue that initiates a specific behavior. This behavior leads to a reward, creating a loop that reinforces the habit over time. For example, the sound of a notification might trigger the habit of checking your phone, with the reward being a sense of connection or distraction. Understanding this cycle is essential for transforming habits, as it reveals the mechanics of how they are formed and maintained.

The first step in habit transformation is identifying the habits you wish to change. This requires honest self-reflection and awareness of the behaviors that no longer serve you. Journaling or tracking your daily actions can help uncover patterns. For instance, you might notice a tendency to procrastinate on tasks by scrolling through social media, or a habit of reaching for unhealthy snacks during stressful moments. Once identified, these habits become opportunities for intentional change.

To transform a habit, start by examining its components: the trigger, the behavior, and the reward. Ask yourself: *What prompts this habit? What need is it fulfilling? What alternative behavior could satisfy this need?* For example, if stress triggers a habit of overeating, the need might be emotional comfort. Replacing this habit with a healthier behavior, such as deep breathing or talking to a friend, addresses the underlying need while breaking the cycle of the old habit.

Setting clear and specific goals enhances the process of habit transformation. Rather than vague intentions like *"I'll exercise more,"* define actionable and measurable objectives: *"I'll go for a 30-minute walk every morning at 7 a.m."* This clarity reduces ambiguity and creates a roadmap for success. Pairing the new habit with an existing routine—known as habit stacking—further reinforces consistency. For instance, adding stretching exercises immediately after brushing your teeth links the new behavior to an established pattern.

The environment plays a significant role in shaping habits. Adjusting your surroundings to support your goals removes friction and makes desired behaviors easier to adopt. For example, placing a water bottle on your desk encourages hydration, while keeping unhealthy snacks out of sight reduces temptation. Similarly, creating reminders—such as setting alarms or placing sticky notes in visible locations—reinforces triggers for positive habits.

Breaking negative habits often requires disrupting their triggers. For example, if late-night screen time disrupts sleep, placing devices in another room before bed eliminates the cue. Alternatively, introducing a pause between the trigger and the behavior creates space for intentional decision-making. When the urge to check your phone arises, pausing for a moment to ask yourself, *"Do I really need to do this right now?"* interrupts the automatic cycle.

Consistency is the cornerstone of habit transformation. Repeating a behavior regularly strengthens its neural pathways, turning it into an automatic pattern over time. Start small, focusing on manageable changes that build momentum. For instance, if your goal is to develop a meditation practice, begin with just two minutes a day and gradually increase the duration. These small wins accumulate, creating a sense of achievement and reinforcing motivation.

Rewards are a powerful motivator in habit formation. Associating positive outcomes with new habits enhances their appeal and sustainability. For example, rewarding yourself with a relaxing activity after completing a workout reinforces the connection between effort and gratification. Over time, the intrinsic benefits of the habit—such as improved health or clarity—become their own reward, reducing reliance on external incentives.

Accountability accelerates habit transformation. Sharing your goals with a friend, mentor, or support group creates a sense of responsibility and encouragement. Regular check-ins provide opportunities to celebrate progress, troubleshoot challenges, and adjust strategies. For example, partnering with a friend for morning runs not only makes the habit more enjoyable but also fosters mutual commitment.

Relapses are a natural part of the process and should be approached with compassion rather than self-criticism. If an old habit resurfaces, use it as an opportunity to reflect: *What triggered this lapse? How can I adjust my approach to prevent it in the future?* Viewing setbacks as learning experiences rather than failures fosters resilience and perseverance.

Visualization enhances habit transformation by connecting you with the long-term benefits of your efforts. Imagine yourself fully embodying the habit you wish to adopt—feeling energized after consistent exercise, focused from daily meditation, or confident from improved communication skills. This mental rehearsal reinforces your commitment, making the habit more tangible and motivating.

Over time, transformed habits create a ripple effect, influencing other areas of life. For example, adopting a habit of journaling gratitude each evening might enhance your emotional resilience, improving relationships and decision-making. These positive cycles compound, creating momentum for ongoing growth and transformation.

The benefits of habit transformation are profound and far-reaching. By aligning daily actions with your values and goals, you create a life of intentionality and purpose. Relationships flourish as consistent habits of communication, empathy, and support strengthen connections. Professionally, habits of focus, discipline, and creativity enhance productivity and innovation. Most importantly, transformed habits empower you to live authentically, aligning your inner world with your external actions.

Ultimately, habit transformation is not just about changing behaviors but about shaping the person you wish to become. Each small, deliberate change contributes to a larger vision of yourself, turning aspirations into reality. Through this practice, you discover that transformation is not a single act but a continuous process of refinement, growth, and empowerment.

In mastering the art of habit transformation, you unlock the ability to create lasting change, one step at a time. Each new habit becomes a building block, constructing a life of alignment, purpose, and fulfillment. By embracing this practice, you take control of your journey, shaping not only your actions but also the person you are becoming.

Chapter 37
Expanding Perception

Perception shapes reality. It determines how we interpret the world, respond to experiences, and interact with others. Yet, perception is not fixed—it is influenced by beliefs, emotions, and experiences, often creating a narrow lens through which we see life. Expanding perception is the practice of broadening this lens, cultivating the ability to see beyond biases, assumptions, and limitations. This process opens new pathways for understanding, decision-making, and transformation, allowing us to engage with the world in richer and more meaningful ways.

The foundation of expanding perception is awareness. Recognizing that our view of the world is subjective, shaped by personal experiences and mental filters, is the first step. These filters include cultural norms, past experiences, and emotional states, all of which influence how we interpret situations. For example, a person with a belief that *"People are untrustworthy"* may view neutral interactions with skepticism, limiting their ability to form meaningful connections. Awareness of these filters invites curiosity about alternative perspectives.

Mindfulness enhances this awareness. By observing thoughts, emotions, and reactions without judgment, mindfulness creates space to question habitual patterns of perception. For instance, if you find yourself reacting defensively to criticism, mindfulness allows you to pause and explore the underlying assumptions driving that reaction: *Am I assuming the feedback is an attack? Could it be an opportunity to grow?* This reflective practice expands your capacity to see situations more objectively.

Challenging assumptions is a powerful tool for broadening perception. Assumptions often operate unconsciously, shaping how we interpret events and interactions. For example, assuming someone's silence during a conversation indicates disinterest may overlook the possibility that they are simply thoughtful or shy. To challenge assumptions, ask yourself: *What evidence supports this belief? What other explanations could exist?* This questioning mindset creates room for alternative interpretations.

Perspective shifting deepens this process. By intentionally viewing situations from different angles, you gain a more holistic understanding. One effective technique is the "three positions" exercise in Neuro-Linguistic Programming (NLP). First, consider the situation from your perspective (Position 1). Next, imagine the perspective of another person involved (Position 2), considering their feelings, motivations, and challenges. Finally, adopt an objective, observer's viewpoint (Position 3), imagining how an uninvolved third party might view the situation. This exercise reduces bias and fosters empathy, helping you navigate complex interactions with greater clarity.

Expanding perception also involves embracing diversity. Engaging with people from different backgrounds, cultures, and perspectives enriches understanding and challenges preconceived notions. For example, learning about another culture's traditions or values can reveal new ways of thinking and being. Conversations with individuals who hold differing opinions—when approached with respect and openness—foster growth and mutual understanding.

Curiosity is a key driver of expanded perception. Cultivating a mindset of curiosity—asking questions, seeking knowledge, and exploring new experiences—broadens the boundaries of what you know and understand. For instance, reading books, attending workshops, or exploring unfamiliar environments stimulates new ideas and perspectives. This practice nurtures intellectual flexibility, enabling you to adapt to change and solve problems creatively.

Visualization is another technique for expanding perception. By imagining scenarios from multiple angles, you train the mind to consider possibilities beyond immediate impressions. For example, visualizing a challenging conversation from both your perspective and the other person's fosters empathy and prepares you for constructive dialogue. This practice sharpens the ability to anticipate and respond to diverse viewpoints effectively.

Emotions play a significant role in shaping perception. Strong emotions, such as fear or anger, can narrow focus, creating a tunnel vision that excludes alternative perspectives. Learning to regulate emotions through techniques like deep breathing, mindfulness, or journaling restores balance, allowing for a more expansive view. For example, pausing to calm yourself after receiving negative feedback enables you to assess its validity and potential value, rather than reacting defensively.

Language also influences perception. The words we use frame our experiences and interactions. For instance, describing a challenge as a "problem" might evoke frustration, while framing it as an "opportunity" inspires creativity and action. Reframing language shifts perception, opening new ways of engaging with the world. Practicing positive and empowering self-talk reinforces this shift, fostering a mindset of possibility and growth.

Nature offers a profound way to expand perception. Immersing yourself in natural environments—whether hiking in the mountains, walking by the ocean, or simply observing a park—broadens awareness and reduces mental clutter. The vastness and beauty of nature provide perspective, reminding us of life's interconnectedness and encouraging reflection on our place within it.

Practices like meditation further enhance perceptual flexibility. Meditation quiets the mind, reducing the noise of habitual thoughts and creating space for new insights. Techniques such as open awareness meditation, where you observe thoughts and sensations without attachment, foster a sense of openness and curiosity about life's complexities.

Expanding perception also benefits relationships. By seeking to understand others' viewpoints, you strengthen connections and build trust. For example, during a disagreement, actively listening to the other person's perspective—rather than preparing a rebuttal—creates a foundation for resolution. This practice fosters empathy, allowing you to navigate conflicts with greater understanding and compassion.

Professionally, expanded perception enhances decision-making and innovation. Leaders who cultivate diverse perspectives within teams harness a wealth of ideas and solutions, driving creativity and success. For example, brainstorming sessions that encourage input from individuals with varied expertise and backgrounds generate richer and more effective outcomes.

The journey of expanding perception is ongoing, requiring continuous effort and openness. Regular reflection—through journaling, conversations, or mindfulness—helps integrate new perspectives into daily life. Celebrating moments of insight and growth reinforces the practice, motivating further exploration.

Ultimately, expanding perception transforms not only how you see the world but also how you engage with it. It nurtures a sense of wonder, adaptability, and connection, enriching every aspect of life. By broadening your lens, you unlock the ability to navigate complexity, embrace diversity, and create a future defined by understanding and possibility.

In mastering the art of expanding perception, you discover that the world is far richer and more nuanced than it may first appear. Each new perspective reveals layers of insight, inspiring growth and transformation. Through this practice, you learn to approach life with curiosity, empathy, and openness, unlocking the limitless potential of a mind willing to see beyond its boundaries.

Chapter 38
The Flow of Life

Flow is a state of optimal experience where focus, creativity, and performance merge seamlessly. It is often described as being "in the zone," where time feels suspended, challenges become invigorating, and actions seem effortless yet profoundly effective. The flow of life is more than a fleeting sensation; it is a way of engaging with the world that fosters fulfillment, purpose, and resilience. Understanding and cultivating this state unlocks the potential to live and work with heightened clarity and joy.

Flow is characterized by complete immersion in an activity. In this state, the mind and body work in harmony, unhindered by distraction or self-doubt. It arises when the demands of a task align with an individual's skill level, creating a balance between challenge and capability. For example, an artist painting with full concentration or a runner lost in the rhythm of their strides exemplifies flow.

The first step to accessing flow is identifying activities that naturally evoke this state. Reflect on moments when you felt completely absorbed in what you were doing, whether at work, during a hobby, or in conversation. Ask yourself: *What was I doing? Why did it captivate me?* These moments often hold clues to your unique pathways to flow.

Setting clear goals enhances the likelihood of entering flow. A sense of purpose and direction focuses attention, minimizing the mental clutter that often impedes engagement. For example, breaking a complex project into smaller, well-defined tasks creates a roadmap that encourages progress while maintaining focus. The clarity of "what" you aim to achieve directs the energy and intention necessary to immerse yourself fully.

Eliminating distractions is essential for cultivating flow. The modern world is filled with interruptions—from notifications to environmental noise—that pull attention away from the present moment. Creating a dedicated space for focused work or creative expression supports immersion. For instance, silencing devices, organizing your workspace, and setting boundaries with others signal your intention to fully engage with the task at hand.

Flow thrives on challenge. Tasks that are too easy lead to boredom, while those that are too difficult create frustration. The sweet spot lies in the zone of proximal development, where the task stretches your abilities without overwhelming them. For example, a musician might find flow by practicing a challenging yet attainable piece, gradually increasing its complexity as their skill grows. This balance between effort and capability keeps the mind energized and engaged.

Engagement with the present moment is a cornerstone of flow. Mindfulness practices, such as deep breathing or body scanning, prepare the mind for immersion by grounding it in the now. Before beginning an activity, take a few moments to center yourself, clearing away thoughts of the past or future. For example, a writer might start a session with a brief meditation, focusing on the rhythm of their breath to quiet distractions and open the creative channels.

Intrinsic motivation—doing something for its inherent enjoyment rather than external rewards—is a key driver of flow. Activities that align with your passions and values naturally draw you into a state of deep engagement. For instance, a gardener tending to their plants out of love for nature is more likely to experience flow than someone doing the same task out of obligation. Reflecting on what brings you joy and meaning helps identify opportunities to cultivate this state.

Feedback is integral to maintaining flow. Immediate and clear feedback, whether from the task itself or from external sources, provides a sense of progress and guides adjustments. For example, a video gamer receives constant feedback through game mechanics, which keeps them immersed and motivated. Similarly, a writer reviewing their own words or receiving input from peers can refine their work in real time, sustaining engagement.

The body plays an important role in accessing flow. Physical well-being—adequate rest, nutrition, and movement—supports the energy and focus needed for sustained immersion. Activities that involve physicality, such as sports, dance, or yoga, often provide direct access to flow by aligning movement with mindfulness. For instance, a runner attuned to their breath and stride finds harmony between body and mind, entering a state of effortless focus.

Resilience enhances the ability to return to flow after disruptions. Life's unpredictability often interrupts immersion, whether through external events or internal doubts. Developing resilience through practices like mindfulness, affirmations, or reframing setbacks ensures that interruptions become temporary rather than definitive. For example, a programmer troubleshooting an error can view it as part of the creative process rather than a failure, allowing them to reenter flow with renewed focus.

Over time, cultivating flow transforms not only individual experiences but also the broader rhythm of life. The more frequently you access this state, the more it influences your overall mindset and approach. Challenges are no longer viewed as obstacles but as opportunities for growth. Routine tasks take on a sense of purpose and engagement. Relationships deepen as you bring presence and authenticity to interactions.

Flow also enhances creativity and problem-solving. Immersion allows ideas to surface organically, unencumbered by overthinking or fear of failure. For instance, an artist engrossed in their craft might discover new techniques or perspectives that elevate their work. Similarly, professionals in fields ranging from science to entrepreneurship often cite moments of flow as the source of their most innovative breakthroughs.

Sharing the flow experience with others strengthens connection and collaboration. Whether through teamwork in a professional setting or shared hobbies, engaging in activities that foster collective flow creates a sense of unity and synergy. For example, a jazz band improvising together achieves a shared state of flow, where each musician's contribution enhances the whole. This communal experience deepens relationships and inspires mutual growth.

The benefits of living in the flow of life extend far beyond individual tasks. Physically, it reduces stress and enhances well-being by calming the nervous system and fostering a sense of balance. Emotionally, it cultivates joy, fulfillment, and self-efficacy. Professionally, it boosts productivity, creativity, and satisfaction. Most importantly, it aligns your actions with your authentic self, creating a life of meaning and purpose.

Ultimately, the flow of life is about harmony—between effort and ease, challenge and capability, intention and presence. It is a practice of engaging deeply with what matters, allowing yourself to be carried by the current of your own potential. By embracing flow, you discover that fulfillment lies not in the destination but in the experience of fully living each moment.

In mastering the flow of life, you unlock a state of being where transformation becomes effortless. Each step, each action, becomes an expression of your highest self, guiding you toward a future defined by clarity, creativity, and joy. Through this practice, you connect with the essence of life itself—a rhythm of growth, purpose, and boundless possibility.

Chapter 39
Affirmation Techniques

Words carry immense power. They shape our thoughts, influence emotions, and define how we perceive ourselves and the world. Affirmations—positive, intentional statements that reflect desired beliefs or outcomes—are tools for reshaping the inner narrative and aligning the mind with growth and transformation. When practiced consistently and purposefully, affirmations reprogram the subconscious, turning aspirations into reality.

The foundation of effective affirmations lies in clarity and intention. Vague or generalized statements lack the precision needed to inspire meaningful change. Affirmations must be specific, reflecting not just what you desire but how it aligns with your values and goals. For example, instead of saying *"I want to be successful,"* a clearer affirmation might be: *"I am building a fulfilling career by using my skills to create value."* This specificity strengthens the connection between words and actions, fostering a sense of direction and purpose.

Affirmations are most effective when phrased in the present tense. By stating your aspirations as though they are already true, you signal to your subconscious that these beliefs or outcomes are achievable and real. For example, saying *"I am confident and capable in my work"* creates a stronger psychological impact than *"I will become confident and capable."* This shift anchors the affirmation in the now, bridging the gap between intention and embodiment.

Emotional engagement enhances the potency of affirmations. Simply repeating words mechanically has limited effect; they must resonate deeply and evoke a sense of conviction.

Visualizing the affirmation as a lived reality amplifies its impact. For instance, while affirming *"I am healthy and energized,"* imagine yourself engaging in activities that reflect this state—running through a park, feeling vibrant and strong. Engaging all senses in this visualization reinforces the emotional connection, embedding the affirmation more deeply into the subconscious.

Affirmations should focus on what you want to create, rather than what you wish to avoid. The mind tends to fixate on the content of a statement, whether framed positively or negatively. For example, affirming *"I am calm and centered"* is more effective than *"I am not stressed."* The former emphasizes a desired state, while the latter inadvertently reinforces the concept of stress. Framing affirmations positively redirects energy toward growth and possibility.

Consistency is key to embedding affirmations into the subconscious. Like any habit, repetition strengthens neural pathways, turning affirmations into automatic beliefs. Integrating affirmations into daily routines—such as repeating them during morning meditation, writing them in a journal, or saying them aloud before sleep—ensures regular reinforcement. For example, starting each day with *"I am aligned with my purpose and attract opportunities for growth"* sets a tone of intention and focus.

The practice of writing affirmations amplifies their effectiveness. The act of writing engages the brain more deeply than merely speaking or thinking, creating a tangible connection between thought and reality. Journaling affirmations daily, alongside reflections on progress and gratitude, transforms them into an evolving dialogue with yourself. For instance, pairing an affirmation like *"I am resilient in the face of challenges"* with a journal entry about a recent obstacle fosters self-awareness and confidence.

Affirmations can also be enhanced through creative expression. Incorporating them into art, music, or movement channels their energy into action. For example, designing a vision board with images and affirmations that reflect your goals creates a visual and emotional anchor. Similarly, combining affirmations with rhythmic activities, such as walking or dancing, syncs the mind and body, reinforcing the connection between words and experience.

Mindfulness practices further support affirmations. Before repeating affirmations, grounding yourself in the present moment clears mental clutter and prepares the mind to receive. Deep breathing or a brief body scan creates a receptive state, enhancing the affirmation's impact. For example, pairing the affirmation *"I am peaceful and present"* with mindful breathing deepens its resonance, aligning words with physical sensation.

Affirmations work synergistically with other transformative practices. For instance, combining affirmations with gratitude amplifies positivity and reinforces a sense of abundance. Saying *"I am grateful for the strength and opportunities that guide my growth"* not only affirms resilience but also cultivates appreciation. Similarly, aligning affirmations with visualization techniques, such as imagining your ideal future self, creates a cohesive framework for change.

Feedback loops between actions and affirmations strengthen their efficacy. As you act in alignment with your affirmations, their impact becomes self-reinforcing. For example, affirming *"I am disciplined and focused in my studies"* while consistently dedicating time to learning creates tangible evidence of progress, solidifying the belief. Over time, these actions and affirmations form a cycle of growth, where each reinforces the other.

Affirmations are not limited to individual growth; they also enhance relationships and interactions. Affirming positive qualities in others fosters empathy and connection. For example, saying *"I see the strengths and kindness in those around me"* shifts your focus toward appreciating others, transforming how you engage with them. Similarly, collaborative affirmations—such as team members affirming shared goals—strengthen unity and purpose.

Adapting affirmations to life's changing circumstances ensures their relevance and impact. Periodically revisiting and revising affirmations to reflect current goals and challenges keeps them aligned with your journey. For instance, during a career transition, affirmations like *"I am confident in navigating change and discovering new opportunities"* provide support and focus. This adaptability ensures that affirmations remain a dynamic tool for growth.

The cumulative effects of affirmations extend beyond immediate outcomes. Over time, they reshape your self-concept, fostering a mindset of possibility and resilience. Affirmations create a foundation of self-belief, enabling you to approach challenges with confidence and creativity. They also cultivate a sense of agency, reminding you of your ability to influence your thoughts, emotions, and actions.

Ultimately, affirmations are a bridge between who you are and who you aspire to be. They align your inner dialogue with your highest intentions, creating a pathway to transformation. By mastering affirmation techniques, you unlock the power of language to shape your reality, turning dreams into lived experiences.

In embracing the practice of affirmations, you discover that the words you choose have the power to inspire, heal, and empower. Each affirmation becomes a declaration of possibility, a step toward the life you envision. Through this practice, you learn to speak your truth with intention, creating a future guided by clarity, purpose, and unwavering belief in your potential.

Chapter 40
Assertive Communication

Communication is the foundation of human connection, shaping relationships, resolving conflicts, and conveying thoughts and emotions. Among its many forms, assertive communication stands out as a powerful tool for expressing needs, boundaries, and opinions clearly and respectfully. It balances confidence with empathy, ensuring that your voice is heard without overshadowing others. Developing assertive communication transforms interactions, fostering trust, collaboration, and self-assurance.

Assertive communication lies at the midpoint between two extremes: passivity and aggression. Passive communication often avoids conflict but sacrifices self-expression, leading to frustration or resentment. Aggressive communication prioritizes one's needs at the expense of others, often creating tension or alienation. Assertiveness, however, strikes a balance—it advocates for oneself while respecting others, promoting harmony and mutual understanding.

The foundation of assertive communication is self-awareness. Understanding your needs, values, and boundaries provides clarity on what you want to express. Ask yourself: *What do I hope to achieve in this conversation? What emotions or concerns need to be addressed?* This reflection grounds your message in authenticity and purpose. For instance, expressing a concern about workload might stem from a desire for balance and recognition, guiding how you frame the discussion.

Confidence is a cornerstone of assertive communication. This does not mean projecting superiority or dominance but trusting your right to express yourself. Replacing self-doubt with affirmations like *"My perspective is valid and worth sharing"* cultivates the inner assurance needed to communicate effectively. Body language supports this confidence—maintain a relaxed posture, steady eye contact, and a calm tone to convey self-assuredness.

Clarity is essential when communicating assertively. Vagueness or ambiguity can lead to misunderstandings or weaken the impact of your message. Use specific, direct language to articulate your needs or concerns. For example, instead of saying *"I feel like things aren't fair,"* specify the issue: *"I've noticed that I've taken on additional tasks this week, and I'd like to discuss how we can distribute responsibilities more evenly."* This precision enhances understanding and encourages constructive dialogue.

The use of "I" statements is a hallmark of assertive communication. These statements focus on your feelings and needs rather than placing blame or making accusations. For instance, saying *"I feel overwhelmed when deadlines change without notice"* is more effective and less confrontational than *"You're always making last-minute changes."* "I" statements encourage empathy and reduce defensiveness, fostering a collaborative atmosphere.

Listening is as vital to assertive communication as speaking. Active listening—paying full attention, reflecting on what is said, and responding thoughtfully—demonstrates respect and openness. For example, paraphrasing someone's concern—*"I hear that you're feeling frustrated about the timeline"*—validates their perspective, building trust and rapport. This mutual respect creates a foundation for resolving conflicts and finding solutions.

Boundary-setting is a critical skill in assertive communication. Boundaries define what is acceptable and protect your emotional and mental well-being. Expressing boundaries assertively involves clear, respectful language. For instance, if a colleague frequently interrupts your work, you might say: *"I value our discussions, but I need uninterrupted time to focus.*

Could we schedule a specific time to talk?" This approach respects both your needs and the relationship.

Managing emotions is key to maintaining assertiveness, especially in challenging conversations. Strong emotions like anger or frustration can cloud judgment or escalate tension. Techniques such as deep breathing, pausing before responding, or silently affirming your intent to stay calm help regulate emotions. For instance, if you feel provoked during a discussion, taking a moment to center yourself ensures that your response remains constructive.

Assertive communication also involves recognizing and addressing nonverbal cues. Your tone, facial expressions, and gestures often convey as much as your words. For example, maintaining a calm tone reinforces confidence, while an open posture signals approachability. Similarly, observing others' nonverbal cues—such as crossed arms or averted gaze—provides insights into their feelings, guiding how you respond.

Practicing assertiveness in low-stakes situations builds confidence for more challenging interactions. For example, expressing a preference when choosing a restaurant or voicing an opinion in a casual discussion strengthens the habit of assertive expression. As you gain comfort, apply these skills to more significant conversations, such as requesting support at work or addressing conflicts in personal relationships.

Role-playing scenarios with a trusted friend or mentor enhances assertive communication skills. Practicing how to express needs, set boundaries, or handle objections prepares you for real-life situations. Feedback from your practice partner offers insights into your tone, clarity, and body language, helping you refine your approach.

Assertiveness extends beyond individual interactions to create a broader culture of respect and collaboration. Modeling assertive behavior in group settings—such as team meetings—encourages others to communicate openly and constructively. For example, acknowledging diverse perspectives while confidently expressing your own sets a tone of inclusivity and confidence.

Overcoming the fear of assertiveness is a common challenge, particularly for those accustomed to passive or aggressive communication styles. Start small, focusing on one area of your life where assertiveness feels attainable. Celebrate progress, no matter how minor, to build momentum and reinforce your commitment to change. For instance, successfully setting a boundary with a colleague might inspire you to address more complex dynamics in personal relationships.

The benefits of assertive communication ripple across all areas of life. Professionally, it enhances leadership, negotiation, and conflict resolution skills, fostering respect and collaboration. Personally, it deepens relationships, as open and honest communication strengthens trust and understanding. Most importantly, assertiveness empowers you to live authentically, ensuring that your voice and values are fully expressed.

Ultimately, assertive communication is not about controlling conversations but about creating mutual understanding and respect. It is a practice of balancing self-expression with empathy, navigating interactions with confidence and care. By mastering assertive communication, you transform how you connect with others, unlocking the potential for deeper relationships, effective collaboration, and personal empowerment.

In embracing assertive communication, you discover that your voice is a powerful instrument for change. Each word becomes a declaration of your truth, guiding your interactions with clarity and purpose. Through this practice, you learn to navigate the complexities of human connection with confidence, authenticity, and grace, shaping a life enriched by meaningful relationships and effective self-expression.

Chapter 41
Time as an Ally

Time is one of life's most finite and precious resources. How we perceive and utilize it profoundly affects our growth, productivity, and fulfillment. When treated as an adversary, time becomes a source of stress, leading to procrastination or overwhelm. However, when embraced as an ally, it transforms into a tool for achieving goals, living intentionally, and finding balance. Shifting from a reactive to a proactive relationship with time empowers us to align our actions with our values and aspirations.

The first step in making time an ally is reframing how you perceive it. Many people experience time as a scarcity, constantly feeling as though there is never enough. This mindset fosters anxiety and inefficiency. Instead, adopting an abundance mindset—recognizing that time, when used wisely, is sufficient—creates a sense of empowerment. Reflect on your beliefs about time: *Do I view it as something I control, or something that controls me?* Shifting this narrative opens the door to intentional time management.

Understanding your priorities is essential to aligning time with your goals. Without clarity, it's easy to fall into the trap of busyness—filling days with tasks that feel urgent but lack meaningful impact. Begin by identifying your core values and long-term objectives. Ask yourself: *What truly matters to me? How do my daily actions reflect these priorities?* For example, if fostering relationships is a key value, dedicating uninterrupted time to loved ones becomes a non-negotiable aspect of your schedule.

Effective time management requires creating structure while allowing for flexibility. A well-designed plan provides direction without becoming overly rigid. Techniques like time blocking—allocating specific periods for focused work, rest, and recreation—help maintain balance. For instance, reserving mornings for deep work and afternoons for collaborative tasks optimizes energy and focus. Flexibility within this structure accommodates life's unpredictability, ensuring adaptability without derailing progress.

The concept of energy management complements time management. Not all hours are equal; energy levels fluctuate throughout the day. Identifying your peak performance periods allows you to align demanding tasks with high-energy times. For example, if creativity flows best in the evening, reserve that time for brainstorming or problem-solving. By matching tasks to energy levels, you maximize productivity while minimizing burnout.

Eliminating time-wasters is a critical aspect of making time an ally. Distractions—whether in the form of excessive screen time, unnecessary meetings, or multitasking—erode focus and efficiency. Begin by conducting a time audit, tracking how you spend your hours over a week. This exercise reveals patterns and highlights areas for improvement. For example, reducing time spent on social media might free up space for meaningful activities, such as learning a new skill or pursuing a passion.

The practice of prioritization helps distinguish between tasks that are urgent, important, or neither. Tools like the Eisenhower Matrix categorize tasks into four quadrants: urgent and important, important but not urgent, urgent but not important, and neither. This framework clarifies where to focus energy, ensuring that critical long-term goals are not overshadowed by short-term distractions. For instance, scheduling time for professional development, even when not immediately pressing, supports sustained growth.

Procrastination often arises from fear, perfectionism, or lack of clarity. Addressing these underlying causes transforms procrastination into action. Break large tasks into smaller, manageable steps, reducing the intimidation factor. For example, instead of planning to "write a book," commit to drafting one page per day. Celebrating small victories reinforces momentum, turning progress into a consistent habit.

Boundaries play a vital role in protecting your time. Saying no to requests or commitments that conflict with your priorities ensures that your schedule reflects your values. For example, declining an invitation to an event that drains energy or detracts from a critical project preserves time for what truly matters. Communicating boundaries assertively, such as *"I'd love to help, but I'm focusing on other commitments right now,"* reinforces respect for your time.

Mindfulness enhances your relationship with time by grounding you in the present moment. Often, stress about time stems from dwelling on the past or worrying about the future. Practices like meditation, deep breathing, or simply pausing to appreciate the present recalibrate your focus. For instance, dedicating five minutes to mindfulness before starting a task reduces mental clutter, fostering clarity and efficiency.

The art of delegation amplifies your ability to manage time effectively. Delegating tasks that others can handle frees up space for activities that align with your strengths and priorities. For example, outsourcing routine chores or administrative tasks allows you to focus on strategic goals or personal growth. Delegation is not about relinquishing responsibility but about optimizing resources for collective success.

Rest and recovery are essential components of time management. While it may seem counterintuitive, taking regular breaks enhances productivity and creativity. Techniques like the Pomodoro Method—working for a set period (e.g., 25 minutes) followed by a short break—prevent burnout and maintain focus. Similarly, prioritizing sleep, exercise, and relaxation ensures sustained energy and well-being.

Reflection and adjustment keep your relationship with time dynamic and effective. Regularly reviewing your schedule and progress helps identify what's working and what needs to change. For instance, if certain activities consistently feel draining or unproductive, consider eliminating or restructuring them. Reflection also reinforces gratitude for the time spent on meaningful pursuits, strengthening your commitment to intentional living.

Ultimately, time as an ally is about alignment—ensuring that how you spend your hours reflects who you are and who you aspire to be. It transforms time from a constraint into a canvas, allowing you to design a life of purpose, balance, and fulfillment.

In mastering the art of managing time, you unlock the ability to navigate life with clarity and intention. Each moment becomes an opportunity to grow, connect, and contribute, creating a future defined by progress and harmony. By treating time as a trusted partner, you discover that it is not about having more hours in the day but about making each hour count. Through this practice, you reclaim control of your journey, shaping a life that honors your values and aspirations.

Chapter 42
The Practice of Silence

Silence is often overlooked in a world filled with noise, urgency, and constant connection. Yet, it holds transformative power, offering clarity, introspection, and renewal. The practice of silence is not merely the absence of sound but an active engagement with stillness, a space where the mind can rest, creativity can flourish, and deeper truths can emerge. Cultivating moments of silence in daily life fosters self-awareness, emotional balance, and a profound connection to the present moment.

At its essence, silence creates a pause—a break from the relentless flow of thoughts, words, and external stimuli. This pause allows for reflection and grounding, essential elements of personal transformation. Many ancient traditions recognize the value of silence, from meditation practices to periods of solitude observed in spiritual retreats. These practices are not about withdrawal but about recalibration, aligning inner and outer worlds.

The first step in the practice of silence is creating intentional space for it. Modern life often prioritizes activity and productivity, leaving little room for stillness. Identifying moments in your day where silence can naturally fit—such as early mornings, commutes, or evenings—helps establish a routine. For instance, beginning each day with five minutes of quiet contemplation sets a tone of mindfulness and focus.

Mindfulness meditation is a powerful tool for experiencing the benefits of silence. By sitting in stillness and observing the breath, you cultivate awareness of the present moment. Thoughts may arise, but the practice involves gently returning focus to the breath, creating a sense of calm and clarity. For example, during a stressful workday, a brief silent meditation can reset your mindset, improving focus and decision-making.

Nature offers a profound avenue for silence. Immersing yourself in natural settings—walking in a forest, sitting by a river, or watching the sunrise—provides a sensory silence that soothes the mind and body. Nature's rhythms remind us of life's simplicity and interconnectedness, offering perspective and renewal. For instance, pausing to listen to the rustling of leaves or the sound of waves can create a moment of profound stillness and presence.

Silence is also a space for self-reflection. In the absence of external distractions, the mind turns inward, exploring thoughts, emotions, and experiences with greater depth. Journaling in silence amplifies this process, allowing insights to surface. For example, reflecting on a challenging situation in quiet solitude often reveals solutions or perspectives that might remain hidden amidst noise and distraction.

The practice of silence deepens emotional awareness. By sitting with emotions in stillness rather than avoiding or suppressing them, you create space for healing and understanding. For instance, during a moment of sadness, allowing yourself to sit quietly with the feeling—acknowledging it without judgment—fosters acceptance and insight. This practice transforms silence into a tool for emotional resilience.

In communication, silence holds transformative potential. Pausing before responding allows for thoughtful, intentional dialogue, reducing reactive or impulsive exchanges. Similarly, allowing silence to exist during conversations creates space for deeper connection. For instance, during a difficult discussion, a moment of shared silence can convey empathy and understanding more powerfully than words.

Silence can also be a creative force. Many artists, writers, and innovators credit moments of stillness as the birthplace of inspiration. Without the noise of external input, the mind has room to wander and explore, generating ideas and solutions. For example, taking a silent walk during a creative block often sparks new perspectives or breakthroughs, as the mind shifts into a relaxed, receptive state.

Digital silence is increasingly important in an era of constant connectivity. Setting aside time to disconnect from screens and notifications creates space for genuine stillness. For instance, implementing a "digital sunset"—turning off devices an hour before bed—cultivates a peaceful transition to rest and enhances overall well-being. This intentional break from technology reduces mental clutter, fostering clarity and focus.

The challenges of silence often stem from discomfort with stillness. Many people associate silence with awkwardness, boredom, or vulnerability, leading to an instinct to fill it with activity or noise. Confronting this discomfort is part of the practice, revealing underlying fears or patterns that can be addressed. For instance, noticing restlessness during silent meditation may uncover a deeper need for relaxation or self-compassion.

Integrating silence into relationships enhances connection and understanding. Shared silence, such as sitting quietly with a loved one, creates a space for presence and intimacy beyond words. For example, a couple practicing silent mindfulness together might find a renewed sense of closeness, as the absence of conversation allows their shared energy to deepen.

Silence as a tool for decision-making provides clarity and focus. When faced with a complex choice, stepping away from noise and sitting in stillness helps untangle thoughts and align decisions with values. For instance, pausing in silence before responding to a significant opportunity allows intuition and reflection to guide your actions.

The practice of silence does not require perfection or prolonged retreats. Small, consistent moments of stillness—whether a few minutes of mindful breathing or a quiet walk in the evening—accumulate, creating profound shifts over time. These moments anchor you in the present, reducing stress and enhancing awareness.

Over time, silence becomes not just a practice but a state of being, woven into daily life. It teaches you to listen—not only to the world around you but to your own inner voice. It cultivates a deeper relationship with yourself and with others, grounded in authenticity and presence.

Ultimately, the practice of silence is a journey inward, reconnecting you with the essence of who you are. It reveals that beneath the noise of life lies a wellspring of wisdom, creativity, and peace. By embracing silence, you discover that stillness is not an absence but a presence—a space where transformation begins, where clarity emerges, and where the flow of life unfolds with grace and purpose.

Through the practice of silence, you learn to navigate life with greater ease and insight. Each pause becomes an opportunity to reset, reflect, and realign, creating a rhythm that supports growth and fulfillment. In this stillness, you find not emptiness but fullness, a quiet power that guides you toward your truest self.

Chapter 43
Perspective Shifting

Perspective shapes how we experience the world. It influences decisions, emotions, and relationships, often acting as the lens through which challenges and opportunities are perceived. While our default perspectives provide stability and understanding, they can also limit our ability to adapt or grow. Perspective shifting—the intentional practice of viewing situations, events, or relationships from multiple angles—unlocks new possibilities, fosters empathy, and enhances problem-solving. It is a vital skill in personal transformation, offering tools to navigate complexity and expand understanding.

Perspective shifting begins with awareness of your current lens. Every perspective is shaped by beliefs, experiences, and emotions, which can create blind spots or biases. For example, interpreting constructive criticism as a personal attack might stem from past experiences of harsh judgment. Recognizing that this interpretation is only one perspective opens the door to exploring others. Ask yourself: *What assumptions am I making? How else could I view this situation?* This curiosity sets the foundation for change.

One powerful tool for perspective shifting is the practice of empathy. Empathy invites you to step into another person's shoes, exploring their feelings, motivations, and challenges. For instance, during a conflict, imagining how the other person perceives the situation helps uncover common ground and fosters resolution. To deepen this practice, consider their background, values, and needs: *What might they be experiencing? Why might they see things differently?* This mental exercise nurtures understanding and reduces defensiveness.

The "perceptual position" technique in Neuro-Linguistic Programming (NLP) offers a structured approach to shifting perspectives. It involves exploring a situation from three distinct viewpoints:

First Position: Your own perspective, focusing on your feelings, goals, and interpretations.

Second Position: The other person's perspective, imagining their thoughts, emotions, and experiences.

Third Position: A neutral observer's perspective, detached from personal involvement, assessing the situation objectively.

By cycling through these positions, you gain a multidimensional understanding of the situation, clarifying emotions, intentions, and potential solutions. For example, in a workplace disagreement, viewing the issue from your colleague's perspective and then from a third-party standpoint may reveal overlooked opportunities for compromise.

Perspective shifting also involves embracing diversity of thought and experience. Engaging with people from different cultures, professions, or belief systems challenges your assumptions and broadens your worldview. For instance, reading literature from another culture or participating in discussions with individuals who hold opposing views provides fresh insights, fostering adaptability and creativity. The willingness to seek and value diverse perspectives enriches understanding and builds bridges across differences.

Nature provides a metaphor for perspective shifting. Climbing a mountain offers a literal change in viewpoint, where the higher vantage point reveals patterns and relationships invisible from the ground. Similarly, stepping back from immediate concerns and viewing them from a broader context illuminates underlying dynamics. For example, shifting focus from a single setback to the larger trajectory of personal growth highlights progress and resilience.

Visualization enhances perspective shifting by engaging the imagination. Mentally rehearse seeing a challenge or decision from different angles. For instance, if you feel stuck in a career decision, visualize the outcomes of each option not just from your perspective but also from the impact it might have on others—family, colleagues, or clients. This exercise creates a more comprehensive understanding, informing choices that align with your values and goals.

Perspective shifting is particularly powerful in overcoming limiting beliefs. These beliefs often narrow your view of what is possible, creating self-imposed barriers. For example, the belief *"I'm not creative"* might limit your willingness to explore new ideas. Challenging this perspective involves asking: *What evidence supports this belief? What counterexamples exist?* Reframing the belief—*"Creativity takes practice, and I'm willing to learn"*—opens new pathways for growth.

In relationships, perspective shifting fosters empathy and reduces conflict. Misunderstandings often arise when each person clings to their own viewpoint, unable to see the other's perspective. Practicing active listening—focusing fully on the other person's words, tone, and body language—creates space for mutual understanding. For example, during a disagreement, reflecting back what you hear—*"It sounds like you're frustrated because you feel unheard"*—validates their experience, building trust and connection.

Perspective shifting is also a tool for navigating uncertainty and change. When faced with unexpected challenges, the default perspective may focus on loss or fear. Intentionally shifting to a growth-oriented perspective—asking *What can I learn from this? How might this create new opportunities?*—reframes the situation, fostering resilience and adaptability. For example, viewing a career setback as a chance to reassess goals and explore new directions transforms adversity into a stepping stone.

Practices like journaling and mindfulness support perspective shifting by creating space for reflection. Journaling prompts such as *What am I not seeing in this situation? How might someone else view this?* encourage exploration of alternative viewpoints. Similarly, mindfulness cultivates detachment from automatic reactions, enabling you to respond with intention rather than habit.

Perspective shifting extends beyond individual growth, shaping how you contribute to collective challenges. Leaders who embrace diverse perspectives within teams foster innovation and collaboration. For example, encouraging team members to share their unique viewpoints during brainstorming sessions creates richer solutions. By valuing and integrating different perspectives, you build environments of inclusivity and creativity.

Over time, perspective shifting becomes a natural and intuitive practice, enriching every aspect of life. It teaches flexibility—the ability to adapt to changing circumstances and see opportunities where others might see obstacles. It deepens relationships, fostering empathy and understanding. Most importantly, it empowers you to approach challenges with curiosity and openness, transforming limitations into possibilities.

Ultimately, perspective shifting reveals that there is no single way to view the world. Every situation, challenge, or relationship holds multiple truths, each offering its own insights and opportunities. By embracing this practice, you unlock the ability to navigate life's complexities with wisdom and grace.

Through perspective shifting, you discover that transformation lies not in changing what you see but in changing how you see. Each new perspective adds depth and dimension to your understanding, creating a fuller, richer experience of life. By cultivating this skill, you align with the endless possibilities of growth, connection, and purpose, navigating your journey with clarity and compassion.

Chapter 44
The Subconscious

The subconscious mind is a vast and powerful force, shaping thoughts, behaviors, and perceptions often without conscious awareness. It stores memories, beliefs, and patterns, acting as a repository of experiences that influence daily life. While its automatic functions can support growth and efficiency, unexamined patterns within the subconscious can also create barriers. Learning to access, understand, and reprogram the subconscious unlocks the potential for profound personal transformation.

The subconscious operates as an intricate system of associations. From a young age, it absorbs information from experiences, emotions, and environmental influences, forming the foundation of beliefs and habits. For instance, a childhood experience of failure might imprint a belief like *"I'm not capable,"* which continues to influence behavior long after the initial event. Identifying and reshaping these subconscious patterns is key to creating new possibilities.

Accessing the subconscious begins with awareness. It communicates through subtle signals—emotions, dreams, and recurring patterns of thought or behavior. Paying attention to these signals provides clues to what lies beneath the surface. For example, recurring feelings of self-doubt might point to a deeply held belief about inadequacy. Journaling or mindfulness practices help bring these subconscious patterns into conscious awareness, creating the opportunity for change.

Relaxation techniques are a gateway to the subconscious. When the mind enters a relaxed state—such as during meditation or deep breathing—it becomes more receptive to exploration and reprogramming. Practices like guided visualization or progressive muscle relaxation quiet the conscious mind, allowing access to subconscious thoughts and beliefs. For instance, envisioning a peaceful place during a guided meditation can help uncover hidden fears or desires associated with that imagery.

The use of affirmations is a powerful tool for influencing the subconscious. Repeating positive, intentional statements rewires neural pathways, gradually replacing limiting beliefs with empowering ones. For example, affirming *"I am worthy of success"* helps counteract deeply ingrained doubts. To enhance effectiveness, pair affirmations with visualization—imagine yourself embodying the affirmation, engaging all your senses to make the experience vivid and believable.

Visualization techniques engage the subconscious by harnessing its preference for images over words. The mind responds strongly to mental pictures, interpreting them as real experiences. For example, athletes often use visualization to rehearse performances, mentally practicing movements and scenarios to improve actual performance. Similarly, visualizing yourself confidently handling a challenging situation primes the subconscious for success, aligning thoughts and actions with desired outcomes.

Hypnotherapy is another approach to accessing the subconscious. Guided by a trained practitioner or through self-hypnosis techniques, this practice induces a state of focused relaxation where subconscious patterns can be explored and reshaped. For instance, someone struggling with procrastination might uncover and address the underlying fear of failure through hypnotherapy, creating space for more productive habits.

The language of the subconscious is symbolic, often expressed through dreams or creative processes. Dreams, in particular, offer a window into subconscious thoughts and emotions. Keeping a dream journal allows you to record and interpret these symbolic messages, uncovering insights that may not surface in waking life. For example, recurring dreams of being unprepared might reveal subconscious anxieties about control or competence.

Art and creative expression also tap into the subconscious. Activities like painting, writing, or freeform drawing bypass the analytical mind, allowing subconscious themes to emerge. For instance, journaling freely without censoring thoughts often reveals surprising insights, as the act of writing provides a direct channel to subconscious concerns or desires. Similarly, creating abstract art can evoke feelings or patterns that reflect subconscious states.

Reframing memories is a powerful technique for reprogramming the subconscious. While the events of the past cannot be changed, their emotional impact can be transformed. For example, revisiting a memory of failure and identifying the lessons it offered reframes it as a source of growth rather than limitation. Practices like the Emotional Freedom Technique (EFT), which combines gentle tapping on acupressure points with affirmations, further support this reframing process by releasing emotional blockages tied to past experiences.

The subconscious thrives on repetition. Patterns repeated over time solidify into automatic behaviors and beliefs. To create lasting change, it is essential to consistently reinforce new patterns. For instance, establishing a daily habit of gratitude journaling rewires the subconscious to focus on abundance and positivity. Similarly, repeatedly practicing a new skill or behavior strengthens neural connections, embedding it into the subconscious as second nature.

Understanding the subconscious also involves recognizing its protective role. Many limiting beliefs or behaviors are rooted in the subconscious's attempt to safeguard well-being. For example, procrastination might stem from a fear of criticism, as the subconscious seeks to avoid potential failure. Approaching these patterns with compassion rather than judgment fosters a collaborative relationship with the subconscious, enabling gentle and effective transformation.

Connecting with the subconscious enhances decision-making and intuition. The subconscious processes vast amounts of information, often detecting patterns and insights that the conscious mind overlooks. Practices like meditation, dreamwork, or simply pausing to reflect on a "gut feeling" enhance access to this intuitive wisdom. For example, pausing to tune into your intuition when faced with a difficult choice often reveals a clarity rooted in subconscious processing.

Over time, working with the subconscious creates alignment between conscious goals and underlying beliefs. This alignment eliminates internal conflicts, where conscious desires are undermined by subconscious doubts. For example, aligning a conscious goal of career success with a subconscious belief in your capability creates a unified focus, enhancing motivation and effectiveness.

The benefits of accessing and reprogramming the subconscious extend beyond individual growth. Relationships improve as subconscious patterns—such as fears of vulnerability or unmet needs—are addressed and transformed. Professional success flourishes as limiting beliefs about ability or worthiness are replaced with confidence and clarity. Most importantly, engaging with the subconscious deepens self-awareness, creating a life rooted in authenticity and purpose.

Ultimately, the subconscious is not a mysterious force to be feared but a powerful ally in transformation. By understanding its role, communicating with it effectively, and reshaping its patterns, you unlock the potential to create the life you envision. The subconscious becomes a partner in growth, aligning your inner world with your outer actions.

Through the practice of engaging with the subconscious, you discover that change begins from within. Each belief reexamined, each pattern reshaped, creates a ripple effect of transformation, empowering you to navigate life with confidence and intention. By unlocking the wisdom of your subconscious, you access the limitless potential that lies beneath the surface, guiding you toward your truest self.

Chapter 45
Strengthening Self-Confidence

Self-confidence is the foundation of growth and achievement, a quality that empowers individuals to take risks, pursue goals, and navigate challenges with resilience. It is not an innate trait reserved for a select few but a skill that can be cultivated through intentional practice and self-awareness. Strengthening self-confidence involves aligning thoughts, emotions, and actions to build a sustainable belief in one's abilities and worth.

True self-confidence is rooted in self-acceptance—the ability to embrace yourself fully, including your strengths and imperfections. It is not about eliminating doubts or becoming impervious to criticism but about maintaining trust in your capacity to learn, adapt, and overcome. This trust becomes the cornerstone of confident actions, regardless of external circumstances.

Building self-confidence begins with reframing negative self-perceptions. Many people carry inner narratives shaped by past experiences, such as *"I'm not good enough"* or *"I always fail."* These beliefs, often rooted in childhood or moments of vulnerability, can undermine confidence. Start by identifying these limiting thoughts through self-reflection or journaling. Challenge their validity by asking: *Is this belief based on fact, or is it an assumption? What evidence contradicts it?* Replacing these thoughts with affirmations like *"I am capable and growing"* reprograms the mind toward self-assurance.

Action is a powerful catalyst for confidence. Confidence grows not from waiting for perfection but from taking steps, even when fear or uncertainty is present. For example, if public speaking feels daunting, begin by speaking in small, supportive groups. Each success, no matter how small, reinforces the belief in your ability to handle challenges. Over time, these incremental victories create a foundation of self-assurance.

Visualization techniques enhance self-confidence by engaging the imagination to rehearse success. Close your eyes and picture yourself succeeding in a situation that typically evokes doubt. Imagine the sights, sounds, and feelings of this success in vivid detail. For example, if preparing for a job interview, visualize entering the room with poise, answering questions with clarity, and leaving with a sense of accomplishment. Repeated visualization conditions the mind to expect and believe in positive outcomes.

Setting achievable goals builds confidence step by step. Break larger objectives into smaller, manageable tasks that offer regular opportunities for success. For instance, if you aim to improve physical fitness, start with short, consistent workouts rather than attempting an intense regimen immediately. Celebrating these small milestones reinforces progress and fosters a sense of capability.

Positive self-talk is a critical tool for building self-confidence. The language you use to describe yourself influences how you feel and act. Replace self-critical thoughts with empowering statements. For example, transform *"I can't handle this"* into *"I'm learning and improving with every step."* Over time, these shifts in language reshape your inner narrative, aligning it with a confident mindset.

Surrounding yourself with supportive individuals strengthens confidence by providing encouragement and constructive feedback. Seek out relationships that inspire and uplift, avoiding environments that perpetuate doubt or negativity. For example, joining a group of like-minded individuals pursuing similar goals fosters camaraderie and shared growth. Sharing experiences with others also normalizes challenges, reminding you that self-doubt is a universal experience.

Body language influences self-perception and how others perceive you. Adopting confident postures—standing tall, maintaining eye contact, and speaking with a steady tone—sends a signal to your brain that you are capable and in control. For instance, before entering a stressful situation, practicing a "power pose," such as standing with your hands on your hips and feet firmly planted, boosts both psychological and physical confidence.

Learning from failure is a hallmark of self-confidence. Rather than viewing mistakes as evidence of inadequacy, reframe them as opportunities for growth. Ask yourself: *What can I learn from this experience? How can I apply this lesson moving forward?* For instance, if a presentation does not go as planned, identify areas for improvement and focus on refining your approach for the next opportunity. Each failure becomes a stepping stone toward mastery.

Developing competence in specific skills naturally enhances confidence. Investing time in learning, practicing, and refining your abilities builds a sense of expertise and assurance. For example, if writing feels intimidating, taking a course or dedicating time to daily practice builds proficiency and confidence in your abilities. Mastery of one area often spills over into other aspects of life, creating a ripple effect of self-assurance.

Mindfulness practices support confidence by fostering presence and reducing self-critical thoughts. Techniques like meditation, deep breathing, or grounding exercises help quiet the mental chatter that fuels doubt. For example, during a moment of nervousness, focusing on the rhythm of your breath anchors you in the present, allowing you to act with greater clarity and calm.

Embracing your unique strengths reinforces confidence in your individuality. Reflect on qualities, skills, or experiences that set you apart, and consider how they contribute to your goals. For instance, a natural talent for connecting with people might become a cornerstone of your professional or personal success. Recognizing and celebrating these strengths shifts the focus from perceived shortcomings to assets.

Acting "as if" is another strategy for building confidence. Even if self-assurance feels elusive, behaving as though you are confident often leads to genuine feelings of empowerment. For example, walking into a meeting with a purposeful stride and a positive mindset projects confidence, which can influence both your emotions and how others respond to you.

Over time, these practices create a robust and enduring sense of self-confidence. This confidence becomes a foundation for resilience, enabling you to navigate uncertainty and pursue ambitious goals with conviction. It fosters authenticity, allowing you to express yourself fully and engage with the world on your terms.

Ultimately, strengthening self-confidence is about cultivating trust in yourself—trust in your abilities, decisions, and capacity to grow. It is not the absence of doubt but the willingness to move forward despite it, knowing that each step builds strength and wisdom.

Through the practice of self-confidence, you discover that your worth is not determined by external validation but by your own belief in who you are and what you can achieve. This belief becomes a guiding force, empowering you to face challenges, seize opportunities, and live a life defined by courage, authenticity, and purpose.

Chapter 46
The Art of Forgiveness

Forgiveness is one of the most transformative and liberating practices on the journey of personal growth. It is often misunderstood as condoning harm or forgetting the past, but true forgiveness is an act of self-empowerment. It is the conscious decision to release resentment, anger, and pain, freeing yourself from their emotional weight. Through forgiveness, you reclaim your energy, restore inner peace, and create space for healing and renewal.

Forgiveness begins with understanding its purpose. It is not about excusing the behavior of others or invalidating your own feelings but about severing the emotional tether that binds you to the hurt. Holding onto resentment often perpetuates suffering, keeping the wound open and influencing your thoughts and actions. Forgiveness offers a pathway to break this cycle, allowing you to move forward with clarity and grace.

The first step in the art of forgiveness is acknowledging the pain. Suppressing or denying feelings of hurt only deepens their impact. Instead, allow yourself to fully experience and validate your emotions—whether anger, sadness, or betrayal. Journaling about the event or speaking with a trusted confidant provides an outlet for processing these feelings. For example, writing a letter to the person who hurt you (even if it is never sent) allows you to articulate your emotions and gain perspective.

Understanding the context of the situation often facilitates forgiveness. Reflecting on the other person's motivations, limitations, or circumstances does not excuse their actions but fosters empathy. Ask yourself: *What might have driven this behavior? Was it a reflection of their own pain, fear, or insecurity?* For instance, recognizing that someone's harsh words stemmed from their own struggles can soften the intensity of your hurt and create a sense of compassion.

Forgiving yourself is equally essential. Many people carry guilt or shame for past actions, decisions, or perceived failures, creating a barrier to self-acceptance. Self-forgiveness involves acknowledging mistakes, taking responsibility where appropriate, and committing to growth. For example, if you regret a decision that caused unintended harm, reflect on what you have learned and how you can act differently moving forward. Affirmations like *"I release myself from guilt and embrace my ability to grow"* reinforce this process.

Reframing the narrative of the hurtful event transforms its impact. Instead of viewing it solely as a source of pain, consider the lessons or growth it inspired. For example, a betrayal might teach the importance of setting boundaries or trusting your intuition. This shift in perspective does not minimize the pain but integrates it into your story as a catalyst for strength and resilience.

Letting go of resentment often requires conscious effort and time. Visualizations can support this process. Imagine the resentment as a heavy burden you are carrying. Picture yourself gradually releasing it, watching it dissolve or drift away, leaving you lighter and freer. For instance, envision placing the pain into a flowing river, allowing the current to carry it far from you. This mental exercise reinforces your intention to let go.

Boundaries play a crucial role in forgiveness. Forgiving someone does not mean reestablishing the same relationship or tolerating harmful behavior. It is possible to forgive while maintaining boundaries that protect your well-being. For example, you might forgive a friend for their hurtful actions but decide to limit your interactions with them. Forgiveness is about emotional release, not necessarily reconciliation.

Rituals can add a symbolic element to forgiveness, helping to solidify the process. For example, writing down your resentments and then burning or tearing the paper creates a tangible representation of release. Similarly, practices like meditating on forgiveness, lighting a candle, or repeating a mantra—*"I release this pain and open myself to peace"*—anchor the act of letting go in a meaningful way.

Forgiveness is a deeply personal journey that unfolds at its own pace. There is no "right" timeline for letting go of pain, and forcing the process can lead to superficial resolution. Instead, approach forgiveness with patience and compassion, allowing yourself to move through the layers of emotion naturally. For instance, if revisiting the hurt feels overwhelming, focus on small steps, such as acknowledging your desire to forgive without pressuring yourself to achieve it immediately.

Forgiveness also extends to forgiving life itself for its unpredictability or perceived injustices. Many people harbor resentment toward circumstances—such as illness, loss, or failure—that feel unfair or undeserved. Cultivating acceptance of life's impermanence and challenges shifts this perspective, fostering peace and gratitude. Practices like mindfulness or gratitude journaling help reframe these experiences, highlighting the growth and resilience they inspire.

Forgiveness benefits not only the individual but also relationships and communities. When practiced collectively, forgiveness fosters reconciliation and understanding. For example, in the aftermath of a conflict, openly expressing forgiveness can mend trust and restore harmony. Sharing the journey of forgiveness with others—whether through conversation, support groups, or shared rituals—amplifies its transformative power.

The emotional and physical benefits of forgiveness are profound. Releasing resentment reduces stress, anxiety, and tension, creating space for joy and well-being. It strengthens emotional resilience, enhancing your ability to navigate future challenges with grace. Most importantly, forgiveness liberates you from the past, allowing you to live fully in the present.

Ultimately, the art of forgiveness is an act of self-love. It is a gift you give yourself, freeing your heart from the weight of pain and opening it to healing and possibility. Forgiveness does not erase the past but transforms its impact, turning wounds into wisdom and strength.

Through the practice of forgiveness, you discover that peace lies not in changing the past but in changing how you carry it. Each act of forgiveness becomes a step toward freedom, a declaration of your ability to heal and grow. By mastering this art, you align with the transformative power of compassion, creating a life defined by resilience, understanding, and inner harmony.

Chapter 47
Overcoming Procrastination

Procrastination is a common obstacle on the path to personal transformation, a behavior that often masks deeper fears, doubts, or misaligned priorities. While it may appear as mere avoidance, procrastination reveals valuable insights about motivation, habits, and emotional states. Overcoming procrastination involves more than just time management—it requires understanding its roots, reframing its narrative, and building strategies that align action with purpose.

At its core, procrastination is often a response to emotional discomfort. Tasks may feel overwhelming, dull, or fraught with the fear of failure or judgment. For example, postponing a challenging work project might stem from anxiety about not meeting expectations. Recognizing these underlying emotions is the first step in addressing procrastination. Ask yourself: *What am I avoiding? What emotions arise when I think about this task?* Awareness turns procrastination into an opportunity for self-discovery and growth.

Breaking tasks into smaller, manageable steps reduces the intimidation factor. When a goal feels too large or undefined, it becomes easy to delay action. Dividing it into concrete, actionable pieces creates a sense of progress and momentum. For instance, instead of aiming to "write an entire report," set a goal to "draft an outline" or "write the introduction." Completing these smaller steps builds confidence, making the larger task feel more achievable.

The "two-minute rule" is a practical tool for tackling procrastination. This strategy involves starting any task that takes less than two minutes immediately or dedicating just two minutes to begin a larger task. For example, opening a document and writing a single sentence often leads to continued work, as initiating action reduces resistance. Momentum gained in those initial moments often carries you forward.

Understanding the role of perfectionism in procrastination is key to overcoming it. Perfectionism creates unrealistic standards, making tasks feel insurmountable. For example, delaying a creative project because it might not be "good enough" reflects a fear of imperfection. Reframing perfectionism with a mindset of experimentation—*"Done is better than perfect"*—encourages action over stagnation. Viewing mistakes as opportunities to learn further reduces the fear of starting.

Mindfulness practices help address the emotional resistance behind procrastination. By observing thoughts and emotions without judgment, mindfulness creates space between impulse and action. For instance, noticing the urge to check social media instead of working allows you to pause and choose a more intentional response. Techniques such as deep breathing or grounding exercises calm the mind, making it easier to focus.

Visualizing success enhances motivation by connecting tasks to their desired outcomes. Imagine the benefits of completing a task—how it will feel to achieve the goal, the rewards it will bring, and the stress it will alleviate. For example, visualizing yourself confidently presenting a completed project reinforces the purpose behind the effort, motivating you to take action.

Accountability transforms procrastination into progress. Sharing your goals with a friend, mentor, or group creates a sense of responsibility and support. For instance, agreeing to check in with a colleague about a project milestone encourages follow-through. External accountability complements internal motivation, providing encouragement and perspective.

Eliminating distractions from your environment minimizes opportunities for procrastination. Identify and address common sources of distraction, such as clutter, notifications, or multitasking. For example, dedicating a specific workspace to focused tasks or using apps that block distracting websites reinforces concentration. Structuring your environment to support productivity reduces friction, making it easier to begin and sustain effort.

The role of self-compassion in overcoming procrastination cannot be overstated. Harsh self-criticism often exacerbates avoidance, creating a cycle of guilt and inaction. Instead, approach procrastination with curiosity and kindness: *What might I need right now to move forward?* Replacing self-judgment with encouragement—*"It's okay to struggle; I'm making progress one step at a time"*—fosters resilience and motivation.

Time-blocking techniques structure your day to prioritize important tasks. Allocating specific periods for focused work ensures that critical activities receive attention. For instance, dedicating the first hour of the morning to high-priority tasks capitalizes on peak energy levels and reduces the likelihood of delay. Pairing time blocks with breaks, such as using the Pomodoro Technique, maintains productivity without burnout.

Identifying your peak performance periods aligns tasks with your natural rhythms. For example, if you feel most energized in the morning, reserve that time for challenging or creative work. Understanding when you work best allows you to plan effectively, maximizing both efficiency and satisfaction.

Reconnecting with your "why" provides clarity and motivation. Procrastination often arises when tasks feel disconnected from your values or goals. Reflecting on the larger purpose behind the task—*Why does this matter? How does this align with my aspirations?*—infuses it with meaning. For example, viewing a tedious report as a step toward career advancement transforms it from an obligation into an opportunity.

Procrastination is often fueled by the belief that action requires motivation. In reality, action often precedes motivation. Taking even a small step creates momentum, which generates the motivation to continue. For instance, starting a workout with just a five-minute walk often leads to completing the full session.

Embracing this "action-first" mindset reduces reliance on fleeting motivation.

Rewarding yourself for completing tasks reinforces positive behavior. Pairing effort with enjoyment creates a cycle of progress and reward. For example, treating yourself to a favorite activity after completing a challenging project reinforces the association between effort and satisfaction. These small rewards sustain motivation and make the process more enjoyable.

Overcoming procrastination is a journey of self-awareness and empowerment. It involves shifting from avoidance to intentionality, transforming obstacles into opportunities for growth. By addressing the underlying emotions, breaking tasks into actionable steps, and aligning actions with values, you create a framework for sustained progress.

Ultimately, procrastination is not a reflection of laziness or incapacity but an invitation to understand and realign your relationship with action. Through this practice, you develop resilience, discipline, and clarity, empowering yourself to face challenges with confidence and purpose.

In mastering the art of overcoming procrastination, you discover that progress is built not on perfection but on persistence. Each step forward, no matter how small, brings you closer to your goals, transforming hesitation into momentum and potential into achievement. By embracing this practice, you unlock the power to create, grow, and thrive.

Chapter 48
Celebrating Achievements

Celebrating achievements is a powerful and often overlooked aspect of personal transformation. In the relentless pursuit of goals, it's easy to focus on what remains undone, bypassing the milestones that mark progress. Yet, acknowledging and celebrating achievements fosters motivation, reinforces self-worth, and strengthens the connection between effort and outcome. It transforms the journey of growth into one of joy and fulfillment.

The practice of celebrating achievements begins with recognizing their value, no matter how small. Every step forward contributes to the larger picture of transformation. Whether it's completing a major project, overcoming a fear, or making a small habit change, each accomplishment deserves acknowledgment. Reflect on your recent efforts: *What have I achieved that I haven't yet celebrated?* This awareness shifts focus from what's lacking to what's been gained.

One of the most impactful ways to celebrate achievements is through reflection. Taking time to pause and consider what the accomplishment represents—the challenges overcome, the skills developed, or the growth achieved—deepens its significance. Journaling about these reflections provides a tangible record of progress, which can serve as a source of inspiration during future challenges. For example, documenting the journey of preparing for and delivering a successful presentation reinforces confidence in your abilities.

Celebrating achievements is not only about reflection but also about sharing. Involving others in your celebrations amplifies their impact and builds a sense of community. Share your successes with trusted friends, family, or colleagues who can join in your joy and acknowledge your efforts. For instance, sharing a promotion or a personal breakthrough with loved ones strengthens bonds and creates shared moments of pride and gratitude.

Creating rituals for celebration adds a layer of intention and meaning. Rituals can be as simple as lighting a candle, enjoying a favorite meal, or taking a moment of silence to honor your progress. These practices create a sense of occasion, elevating the act of celebration beyond a fleeting acknowledgment. For example, setting aside time each month to review and celebrate achievements fosters a habit of gratitude and self-recognition.

Rewards are a tangible way to reinforce the connection between effort and achievement. Aligning rewards with personal values and preferences ensures they feel meaningful. For instance, treating yourself to a new book, an experience, or even a day of rest and self-care acknowledges the effort invested in reaching a milestone. These rewards act as positive reinforcement, encouraging continued commitment to your goals.

Celebration is not limited to major achievements. Recognizing small wins creates a consistent pattern of positive reinforcement that fuels motivation. For example, celebrating the completion of a single workout, a productive hour of focused work, or a day of mindful eating reinforces the behaviors that contribute to larger goals. These micro-celebrations sustain momentum and cultivate a sense of ongoing success.

Gratitude is an integral aspect of celebrating achievements. Expressing gratitude for the resources, opportunities, and support that contributed to your success shifts focus from self-criticism to abundance. For instance, after achieving a career milestone, take time to thank mentors, colleagues, or loved ones who played a role in your journey. This practice not only deepens relationships but also fosters a sense of interconnectedness.

Celebrating achievements also involves acknowledging the lessons learned from setbacks or failures along the way. Every challenge faced and overcome contributes to growth. For example, reflecting on how a previous mistake led to the development of resilience or problem-solving skills turns even difficulties into milestones worth celebrating. This perspective fosters a mindset of learning and adaptability.

The way you celebrate reflects your individuality. For some, celebration might involve solitude and introspection, such as meditating on a sense of accomplishment. For others, it might involve social gatherings, creative expression, or physical activity. Tailoring your celebrations to your preferences ensures they feel authentic and meaningful. For example, an artist might commemorate finishing a project by starting a new creative endeavor, while an extrovert might host a small gathering to share their joy.

In professional settings, celebrating achievements enhances morale and fosters a culture of recognition. Acknowledging team successes—whether through a formal event, a shared meal, or a simple thank-you note—creates a sense of shared purpose and motivation. For instance, highlighting individual contributions during a team meeting reinforces the value of collective effort and inspires ongoing collaboration.

Celebration also serves as a pause between milestones, offering a moment of rest and renewal. In the drive to achieve, it's easy to jump from one goal to the next without appreciating the journey. Taking intentional breaks to celebrate creates balance, preventing burnout and restoring energy. For example, after completing a major project, dedicating a weekend to relaxation and enjoyment honors both the effort and the need for self-care.

Over time, the practice of celebrating achievements cultivates a mindset of abundance and positivity. It shifts focus from external validation to internal fulfillment, reminding you that progress is as important as the destination. Each celebration becomes a marker of your growth, reinforcing the belief that you are capable and deserving of success.

Ultimately, celebrating achievements is an act of self-recognition and gratitude. It honors the effort, resilience, and creativity that fuel transformation. By embracing this practice, you transform growth from a relentless pursuit into a joyful journey, one where each step forward is met with acknowledgment and appreciation.

Through the art of celebration, you discover that success is not just about reaching the goal but about valuing the journey. Each milestone becomes a moment to pause, reflect, and rejoice, creating a life enriched by gratitude, pride, and purpose. By mastering this practice, you align with the rhythms of growth, turning every achievement into a source of inspiration and fulfillment.

Chapter 49
Building Connections

Human connections are the lifeblood of personal and collective transformation. Relationships shape how we grow, learn, and experience the world, offering support, perspective, and opportunities for collaboration. Building meaningful and authentic connections is not only a source of fulfillment but also a key driver of resilience, empathy, and shared success. Whether in personal relationships, professional networks, or community engagement, fostering deep and genuine bonds enhances both individual and collective well-being.

Authenticity is the foundation of meaningful connections. True relationships flourish when individuals feel safe to express themselves honestly and without fear of judgment. This begins with self-awareness—understanding your values, boundaries, and emotions—so that you can engage with others from a place of integrity. Ask yourself: *What do I seek in my connections? How can I show up as my true self?* Approaching interactions with authenticity invites others to do the same, creating an atmosphere of mutual trust.

Active listening is a cornerstone of connection. In a world filled with distractions, offering your full attention during a conversation is a powerful act of presence and respect. Practice listening not just to respond but to understand, focusing on the speaker's words, tone, and emotions. For example, when a friend shares a challenge, paraphrasing their feelings—*"It sounds like you're feeling overwhelmed"*—demonstrates empathy and validates their experience.

Empathy deepens relationships by bridging the gap between perspectives. It involves seeing the world through another's eyes, imagining their feelings and experiences. For instance, during a disagreement, pausing to consider the other person's viewpoint—*What might they be feeling? What do they need right now?*—fosters understanding and reduces defensiveness. Empathy transforms conflict into an opportunity for connection and growth.

Vulnerability strengthens bonds by inviting authenticity and trust. Sharing your thoughts, fears, or aspirations with others creates a sense of intimacy, encouraging reciprocal openness. For example, expressing gratitude to a colleague for their support or admitting to a loved one that you're struggling with a decision deepens the relationship by fostering mutual care and understanding. Vulnerability is not weakness but a courageous act that cultivates connection.

Shared experiences are powerful catalysts for building connections. Engaging in activities together—whether collaborative projects, recreational pursuits, or volunteering—creates opportunities for bonding and shared memories. For instance, participating in a team-building retreat or attending a community event provides a space for collective growth and discovery. These shared moments form the basis of lasting relationships, enriched by mutual achievements and experiences.

Effective communication is essential for cultivating connections. Clarity, honesty, and respect in your words foster trust and understanding. Avoiding assumptions, asking clarifying questions, and expressing yourself directly ensure that your intentions align with your actions. For example, instead of saying *"You never listen to me,"* try *"I feel unheard when I'm interrupted, and I'd appreciate it if we could take turns speaking."* This approach promotes constructive dialogue and strengthens the relationship.

Setting boundaries enhances the quality of connections by ensuring that interactions are healthy and respectful. Boundaries define what is acceptable, protecting your emotional well-being while respecting others. For example, if a friend frequently cancels plans last minute, expressing your feelings—*"I value our time together and feel disappointed when plans change unexpectedly. Can we set a time that works for both of us?"*—reinforces your needs while maintaining the relationship.

Networking, often associated with professional settings, is another avenue for building connections. Authentic networking goes beyond exchanging business cards or LinkedIn requests; it's about cultivating genuine relationships based on mutual interest and support. Approach networking with curiosity, focusing on understanding others' goals and offering value. For example, following up after a conference with a note of appreciation or sharing a helpful resource demonstrates sincerity and builds rapport.

Celebrating others' successes strengthens bonds and fosters goodwill. Taking the time to acknowledge a friend's achievement, a colleague's milestone, or a family member's growth reinforces the relationship by showing care and support. For instance, sending a congratulatory message or hosting a small celebration honors their accomplishment while deepening your connection.

In relationships, consistency builds trust and reliability. Regularly showing up for others—whether through check-ins, acts of kindness, or simple presence—demonstrates commitment. For example, a weekly call with a long-distance friend or a habit of supporting a colleague during busy times creates a sense of dependability and care.

Forgiveness is a vital element of connection, allowing relationships to endure challenges and misunderstandings. Holding onto resentment creates distance, while offering forgiveness fosters healing and renewal. For example, after a conflict with a loved one, expressing willingness to move forward—*"I value our relationship and want to work through this together"*—opens the door to reconciliation and growth.

Community engagement expands the scope of connection beyond individual relationships, fostering a sense of belonging and collective purpose. Joining groups, participating in local events, or volunteering with causes that resonate with your values creates opportunities to meet like-minded individuals. For instance, attending a book club or volunteering at a community garden not only strengthens ties with others but also contributes to a greater sense of fulfillment and impact.

Digital connections, when approached mindfully, also play a role in modern relationships. While technology offers convenience, it requires intentionality to ensure meaningful interactions. Focus on quality over quantity, prioritizing thoughtful messages or video calls over superficial exchanges. For example, scheduling a virtual coffee chat with a mentor or sending a personalized message to reconnect with an old friend fosters deeper digital bonds.

Over time, the practice of building connections enriches every aspect of life. Personal relationships become sources of joy, support, and inspiration. Professional networks offer collaboration, learning, and growth. Community ties create a sense of belonging and shared purpose. Each connection contributes to a life of meaning and interdependence.

Ultimately, building connections is about creating spaces where people feel seen, heard, and valued. It is a practice of giving and receiving, of showing up with authenticity and openness. By nurturing these bonds, you create a network of relationships that uplift, inspire, and sustain you.

Through the art of building connections, you discover that transformation is not a solitary journey but a shared experience. Each relationship becomes a mirror, reflecting growth and possibility. By mastering this practice, you align with the power of human connection, creating a life enriched by love, trust, and mutual support.

Epilogue

We have reached the end of a journey that, in truth, never ends. The pages you have traveled through were merely a glimpse, an introduction to the vastness of your potential. But now, as you close this book, the true transformation begins. Because personal alchemy is not a destination but a way of being, a state of continuous evolution.

Reflect on the lessons you have absorbed, on the reflections these words have stirred. They are not final answers but starting points. Transformation is a daily practice, a renewed commitment in every choice, every thought, and every action. What you do with what you have learned here will shape not only your life but also the impact you have on the world around you.

Throughout this reading, you have encountered concepts of profound depth: the power of now, the reconfiguration of beliefs, the reframing of experiences. These elements are more than tools; they are invitations to a more honest inner dialogue, a reconnection with the essence of who you are. It is not about becoming someone different but about peeling back the layers that obscure your authenticity.

And now, as you look at the world, you will notice that it, too, has changed—not because the external reality has shifted, but because you have changed the way you see it. The same situations that once seemed like barriers can now be seen as challenges to be overcome. The same relationships can become fertile ground for growth instead of sources of conflict. This is true alchemy: transforming not only the gold within your soul but everything you touch.

Remember, this journey does not need to be solitary. Every insight you implement, every transformation you experience, reverberates in the people around you. Your evolution is a spark that can ignite others, creating a cycle of collective growth. We are all connected, and your transformation is a contribution to the whole.

As you close this book, do so with gratitude. Not just for what you found here, but for what already existed within you, waiting to be revealed. Every step you took to this moment was essential, and every step you take from here on will be equally significant. You are prepared, equipped, and awakened for what lies ahead.

And finally, remember: the path of personal alchemy does not end. It transforms, just as you do. Keep exploring, questioning, and growing. For life is the great masterpiece, and you, the alchemist.

www.ingramcontent.com/pod-product-compliance
Lightning Source LLC
LaVergne TN
LVHW040054080526
838202LV00045B/3625